"As with the colors in a rainbow, veganism's rewards are infinite and represent the ultimate pot of gold for the billions of land and sea animals who endure the daily thunderstorms wrought by our species. In *Color Me Vegan*, these colors come alive by offering a palette of possibilities for your personal health, for the revival of our planet, and for the now more easily than ever colorfully ethical choices you can make three times a day."

—**Joseph Connelly**, Publisher, *VegNews Magazine*

"Colleen Patrick-Goudreau's recipes are delicious and healthy; but most of all, they are designed with kindness and peace in mind—the very best kind of food for body and soul!"

—**Kathy Freston**, best-selling author of *The Quantum Wellness Cleanse*

"*Color Me Vegan* is a testament to what truly great cuisine is all about: healthful, wholesome ingredients, chosen not only for the pleasure it will give but for the compassion it embodies."

—**Tal Ronnen**, author of *The Conscious Cook*

"Colleen has pulled out the stops with *Color Me Vegan*. This beautiful and informative book contains a treasure trove of plant-delicious recipes. I feel healthier and more energized just looking at this book!"

—**Rip Esselstyn**, bestselling author of *The Engine 2 Diet*

"Blending the latest science on phytonutrients with enticing photos and recipes, this book illumines the many benefits of a cruelty-free kitchen from a fascinating angle: creating artistic dishes based on color. A terrific how-to guide to healthy, delicious, and visually-appealing meals, *Color Me Vegan* could change forever the way you think about food."

—**Dr. Will Tuttle**, pianist, composer, former Zen monk, author of *The World Peace Diet*, and a recipient of the Courage of Conscience Award

"In a world awash in vegan cookbooks, Colleen has come up with another standout that is unique, fun, informative, and compelling!"

—**Matt Ball**, Executive Director of Vegan Outreach and co-author of *The Animal Activist's Handbook*

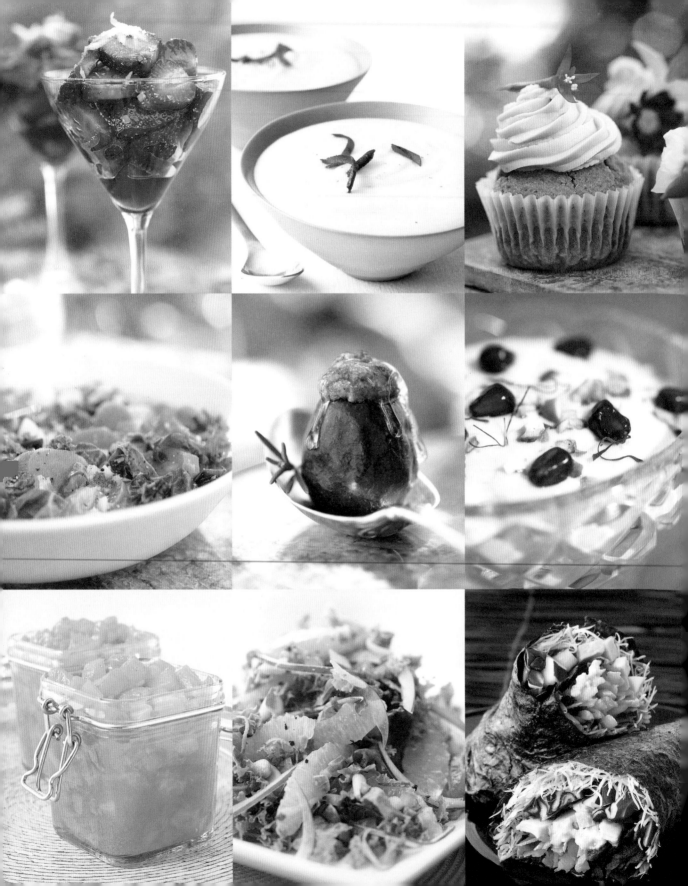

COLOR ME Vegan

Maximize Your Nutrient Intake and Optimize Your Health by Eating Antioxidant-Rich, Fiber-Packed, Color-Intense Meals That Taste Great

COLLEEN PATRICK-GOUDREAU

Author of *The Vegan Table* and the award-winning *The Joy of Vegan Baking*

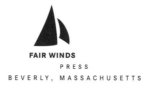

FAIR WINDS
PRESS
BEVERLY, MASSACHUSETTS

Text © 2010 Colleen Patrick-Goudreau
Photography © 2010 Rockport Publishers

First published in the USA in 2010 by
Fair Winds Press, a member of
Quayside Publishing Group
100 Cummings Center
Suite 406-L
Beverly, MA 01915-6101
www.fairwindspress.com

14 13 12 11 10   1 2 3 4 5

ISBN-13: 978-1-59233-439-1
ISBN-10: 1-59233-432-6

Library of Congress Cataloging-in-Publication Data
Patrick-Goudreau, Colleen.
  Color me vegan : maximize your nutrient intake and optimize
your health by eating antioxidant-rich, fiber-packed, color-
intense meals / Colleen Patrick-Goudreau.
     p. cm.
  Includes bibliographical references and index.
  ISBN-13: 978-1-59233-439-1
  ISBN-10: 1-59233-439-3
  1. Veganism. 2. High-fiber diet. 3. Antioxidant. I. Title.
  TX392.P385 2010
  613.2'86--dc22
                              2010028152

Cover and book design: Debbie Berne Design
Photography: Ekaterina Smirnova, all photos unless
                  otherwise noted
                  Bill Bettencourt, pages 47, 63, 97, 114, 127, 136,
                  141, 194, 231, 239, 251
Food Styling: Jen Straus, pages 47, 63, 97, 114, 127, 136, 141,
                  194, 231, 239, 251

Printed and bound in China

To Simon Pieman
You brought color, life, and light into this world,
and it was with dignity, grace, and beauty that you
left it. You are sorely missed and fiercely loved.

CONTENTS

INTRODUCTION

WHY I WROTE THIS BOOK

In the work I do guiding people toward a way of eating that reflects their own compassion and desire for health, I am blessed to hear from countless people whose lives have been transformed. One of the most gratifying responses I receive is from people who've discovered my work because of their interest in eating healthier but who then find that they become open to their compassion for animals. On the flip side, I also hear from people who find my work because of their compassion for animals but who learn to eat healthier. It's so gratifying to fill both these needs.

When it comes to living ethically, my message is simple: live according to your own values of kindness and compassion. When it comes to my message of eating healthfully, my message is equally simple: eat by color.

It really is that easy. When shopping at the grocery store or farmers' market, fill your baskets with color. And when I say color, I mean *naturally occurring* color—not artificial color, not color on a flashy cereal box. I mean the variety of color we admire when walking through a flower garden or strolling through a farmers' market or when imagining an autumn cornucopia. I mean the color in plants. And the healing power of these plants is found in their color.

The Color Is in the Plants

Not that I would do it any other way, but in truth, it would be impossible to write a book on the healthful aspects of colorful foods and include animal products in the form of meat, fish, dairy, or eggs. The only way to authentically write a cookbook that emphasizes the benefits of *eating by color* is to write a vegan cookbook. The phytochemicals, antioxidants, and fiber—all of the healthful components of plant foods—originate in plants, not animals.

Let me repeat: phytochemicals/phytonutrients (*phyto*, after all, means "plant"), antioxidants, and fiber originate in plants, not animals. If they are present, it is because the animal ate *plants*. And why should we go through an animal to get the benefits of the plants themselves? To consume unnecessary, unseemly, and unhealthy substances, such as saturated fat, animal protein, lactose, and dietary cholesterol, is to negate the benefits of the fiber, phytonutrients, vitamins, minerals, and antioxidants that are prevalent and inherent in plants.

Focused on Color

And so with the intention of making it as easy as possible to center your diet around color, I am thrilled to bring you *Color Me Vegan*. Every recipe in this book is guided by color, which enabled me to emphasize the whys and wherefores of eating by color, to encourage you to expand your edible color palette, and to help you increase your health by offering recipes based on nutrient-dense foods. In other words, the organization of this book is meant to raise the bar and give you everything you need to eat consciously, compassionately, and creatively.

Although it was easy to craft so many recipes based on the hundreds of edible plant foods available to us, I made a point to provide as much variety as possible. I also made a conscious effort to keep the recipes simple and the ingredients familiar. I mention some foods that might seem more exotic (purple potatoes, blue cornmeal, and white asparagus), but the fact is these ingredients are more available than ever before in such places as farmers' markets, large natural food stores, and online. But because I'm conscious of ingredients that might be harder to find, I always let you know that the more familiar version may be used in its stead (red potatoes, yellow cornmeal, or green asparagus, respectively).

My hope is that these recipes will help you make nutrient-rich, flavor-dense, aesthetically exciting food choices and that they reflect the abundance of healthful, compassionate options we can make every time we eat.

WHY EAT BY COLOR?

If we've heard it once, we've heard it a thousand times: eat your vegetables! From the day we moved on to solid foods until the day we moved out of the house, we heard this culinary command at least three times a day. Yet at some point, we tuned it out.

A new study confirms this: Americans are eating fewer vegetables than ever. Researchers evaluated data from two large national health surveys and reviewed how many people ate three or more servings of vegetables a day (french fries counted!). In the first survey, 35 percent met the goal; in the second survey, ten years later, only 32 percent did. And as many as 50 percent of Americans don't eat a piece of fruit all day long.

Wisdom of the Ages

Despite the influential role the meat, dairy, and egg industries have on our decisions—not only in terms of market saturation and advertising but also in terms of education materials provided to schools and nutrition policy makers—everyone knows on a basic, instinctive level that we need to consume high amounts of fruits and vegetables.

Even health organizations, which traditionally tend to focus on cure rather than prevention, encourage consumers to eat more fruits and vegetables. The American Heart Association recommends healthy adults "choose five or more servings per day." The American Cancer Society recommends people "eat at least five or more servings of fruits and vegetables each day." The World Cancer Research Fund and the American Institute for Cancer Research report called *Food, Nutrition and the Prevention of Cancer: A Global Perspective* states, "Evidence of dietary protection against cancer is strongest and most consistent for diets high in vegetables and fruits." The National Cancer Institute (NCI) created the "Five-a-Day for Better Health" campaign to promote consumption of these foods.

And these recommendations are based on current research, as if we haven't known this all along. After all, many ancient societies recognized the power of plant foods, both in the East and in the West. Hippocrates, the Greek physician who lived from around 460 to 370 BCE and who is considered the father of Western medicine, said, "Let food be your medicine and your medicine be your food." Pliny the Elder's *Natural History*, an encyclopedia published around 77 to 79 CE, cites the medicinal properties of hundreds of herbs, spices, fruits, and vegetables. Traditional Asian diets are centered around plant foods and have played a huge role in disease prevention.

Changing Habits

So why are we ignoring the messages from health organizations, ancient wisdom, our moms, and our own common sense? Well, I have a few ideas.

Most of us were raised on a meat-centered diet, where vegetables played a minor role and came from a can, were boiled to death, or were drowned in cream sauces and butter. It's no wonder we didn't get hooked on veggies.

We're also ridiculous creatures of habit. Many of us rotate the same dishes over and over, and as the researchers discovered, most people demonstrate very little diversity when choosing vegetables. Here's a secret: when I switched to a plant-based diet, I actually found *more* options. With meat, dairy, and eggs no longer displacing healthful options, a world of plant foods opened up.

One of the most effective ways to make healthful choices every time we eat or shop is to choose foods based on their color, and the most significant characteristic of plant foods is the variety of color. The more colorful your diet, the more varied your diet, and the more plant foods you're eating. And that's a good thing.

Color Concentration

It's a good thing because the foods you'd be reaching for when choosing by color are the very foods that protect us from disease: fruits, vegetables, nuts, seeds, mushrooms, beans, herbs, spices, and whole grains. In other words, you're consuming a *concentration* of healthful properties while eating fewer calories.

There are hundreds of phytochemicals in each of the plant foods we eat. We can detect the highest *concentration*, the highest *saturation* of certain phytochemicals because of their color, such as the blue anthocyanins in blueberries, the orange beta-carotene in carrots, or the red betacyanins in beets, but that doesn't mean these plant foods don't contain other phytochemicals in lower levels. Bananas, for instance, though yellow in appearance, also contain the blue anthocyanin pigments but in lesser amounts. Eating a variety of plant foods ensures that we consume as many phytochemicals as possible.

In other words, even when a single fruit or vegetable is not an all-star source of one particular nutrient or phytochemical, eating an abundance of plant foods means that we accumulate a variety of healthful compounds little by little. The more plant foods we eat and the greater variety we consume means a higher intake of phytochemicals. (See the next section for an explanation of phytochemicals.)

Consuming an assortment of plant foods is also beneficial because it means taking in a *variety* of healthful properties, which affect different parts of our bodies. For instance, lycopene is a phytochemical found in tomatoes, and it concentrates itself in the prostate gland of men. Lutein and zeaxanthin are phytochemicals found in spinach and corn and concentrate themselves in the retina and lens of the eye, contributing to a reduced risk of cataracts and macular degeneration. This is why color *variety* is important.

I have organized this cookbook into eight sections: red, orange, yellow, green, blue/purple, white/tan, brown/black, and rainbow. Just imagine how varied and nutrient-rich your diet would be if you chose to eat from each of these colors each day. Your mother would be proud, your health would improve, and your taste buds would be dancing!

WHAT ARE PHYTOCHEMICALS?

You can't turn around these days without hearing about the benefits of phytochemicals, phytonutrients, or antioxidants. What are these things and why are they so helpful?

Phytochemical and *phytonutrient* are interchangeable words, both of which are built from the Greek word for "plant" (*phyto*). Plants create these chemicals in part to protect themselves from the damage caused by animals, insects, photosynthesis, and UV radiation. More than 900 different phytochemicals have been identified as components of food, and hundreds more are still undiscovered. It is estimated that there may be more than 100 different phytochemicals in just one serving of vegetables.

These phytochemicals protect *us* as much as they protect the plant, and we can easily identify some of them by their color. Phytochemicals/phytonutrients are sometimes actually the *pigments* that give fruits, vegetables, and flowers—all plants—their distinctive hues. Although phytochemicals are not technically classified as nutrients, which are defined as "life-sustaining substances," they have been identified as containing properties associated with disease prevention and treatment, particularly related to the top leading causes of death: cancer, diabetes, cardiovascular disease, and hypertension.

Different phytochemicals play different roles on a molecular level, including reducing cellular damage, preventing cancer cell replication, decreasing cholesterol levels, and causing cancer cells to self-destruct. In the grander scheme, they strengthen the immune system, create healthy blood sugar levels, slow the aging process, keep the brain functioning optimally, and reduce inflammation.

What's the Difference between a Phytochemical and an Antioxidant?

Though they tend to overlap a bit, there *are* differences between a phytochemical and an antioxidant. The best way to distinguish between them is to say that phytochemicals can *act* as antioxidants, but they also play other roles. Antioxidants can be phytochemicals, but they can also be vitamins or minerals. Although most phytochemicals that have been discovered work as antioxidants to promote good health, many of them serve additional functions. The most publicized phytochemicals with antioxidant properties are vitamin C, vitamin E, and beta-carotene (which the body converts into vitamin A). (See the sidebar on page 22 for more on antioxidants.)

Because these substances perform so many beneficial functions, researchers have learned that we need to include a wide variety of plant foods in our meals to get a good supply of antioxidants and a full spectrum of health-protective phytochemicals in our bodies.

Familiar Phytochemicals

My desire in writing this cookbook was to empower people to understand some of the benefits of phytochemicals without getting weighed down in scientific jargon. However, just as "beta-carotene," "lycopene," and "antioxidant" have become household words, I think readers can handle a few more. There are literally hundreds of phytochemicals, so I'm offering only a cursory account of what some scientists have dedicated their lives to, but by the time you've delved into a few recipes, "anthocyanin," "indoles," and "lutein" will be familiar additions to your nutrition and cooking vocabulary.

In no time, you'll become versed in sulforaphanes, carotenoids, and flavonoids. Words such as quercetin, isoflavones, and zeaxanthin will roll off your tongue, and you'll be identifying and admiring the lutein in corn, the curcumin in turmeric, and the crocin in saffron.

At the same time, I don't want people to become obsessed with single nutrients. I think it contributes to our confusion and disempowerment about how to eat well. What I want people to understand is the following:

- Eating a whole foods plant-based diet provides us with an abundance of nutrients to help us attain optimum health.
- These nutrients should be obtained through food—not pills—to experience the full benefits.
- Because phytochemicals originate in plants, every animal product we consume displaces a healthful nutrient-rich plant food we are better off eating.
- Eating a variety of plant foods provides us with a variety of nutrients.

As fun as it is to identify the various pigments/phytochemicals in food, as I do throughout this cookbook, the bottom line is that eating a variety of color provides us with a variety of benefits, and that's a good thing.

HOW TO READ THIS BOOK

Separating the chapters into colors was incredibly gratifying, though I allowed myself some creative license when I needed to shift things around. Hence, Chocolate Cherry Cookies appear in the black/brown chapter but could easily have been added to the red chapter. Cashew and Red Lentil Burgers appear in the white chapter, because of the cashews, but they, too, could have been justifiably placed in the red chapter for the lentils. The idea was to categorize the recipes according to color as best as I could, allowing one color in each dish to take precedence, except in the rainbow chapter, where a variety of colors take center stage.

Eating Outside of the Box

Just as the color choice was fluid, so, too, were some of the decisions about what constitutes a "side dish" versus a "main dish" versus a "salad." Certainly you may switch the dishes around to your liking, making something a "starter" even though it's designated as a "main dish" or serving something as a "side dish" that's in the "salad" category. I'll leave it up to your creativity and preference. Also note that some main dishes are meant for breakfast, though I suppose you can serve Peanut Butter Pancakes (page 210) for dinner if you like!

Clarifying the Oil

My recipes tend to be very low in oil or devoid of oil, though not devoid of whole fat. I do encourage people to make healthful, whole fats part of their diet, but that doesn't mean you always have to cook with oil. When you can cut oil, I recommend you do, though most of the recipes in this book let you decide to sauté in oil versus water. When choosing oils, opt for those that are high in monounsaturated fats and low in polyunsaturated fats. Also, those that have a high smoking point and are mild tasting are also ideal for certain dishes (when you don't want the flavor of the oil to overwhelm the dish). Grapeseed oil matches all of these criteria and is easy to find here in northern California because it is made from the remnants of the wine-making industry (and is thus sustainable because it relies on by-products rather than a fresh crop). Canola, coconut, and olive are my other preferred oils and are interchangeable for the most part, though sometimes I specify a particular oil I think is ideal for that dish.

Sugar Options

When the recipes call for sugar, I specify "granulated sugar," and it generally refers to whatever variation of cane sugar you prefer, whether it is sucanat, turbinado, or white, though the latter is stripped of any nutrients whatsoever. I recommend organic sugar because the growing practices for sugarcane tend to be resource- and pesticide-intensive, affecting both the soil and the people planting and harvesting. Replacing dry sugar for liquid sweeteners (such as agave or brown rice syrup) can be done easily but not without some trial and error (depending on the dish) because it can upset the liquid-to-dry ratio in the recipe.

Go for the Best

Many ingredients have a low-grade and a high-grade version. Sometimes it doesn't matter and sometimes it does. I recommend paying a little extra for "the good stuff." Balsamic vinegar is a good example. Although you can get the cheaper stuff (generally labeled "balsamic vinegar of Modena") for cooking, I highly recommend spending a few extra dollars for the higher-grade balsamic vinegar when its flavor is more prominent, such as in grain, green, and bean salads. You'll find this better vinegar at specialty grocery stores and even farmers' markets.

Yams and Sweet Potatoes

The only vegetable that gives me a headache is the one that is called various things around the country and the world. We don't actually eat true yams in the United States (they grow in Africa and other parts of the world), so when a recipe calls for "garnet" or "jewel" yams, even that's a misnomer. *However*, the general rule is when I call for "yams," I'm referring to the orange-fleshed "garnet" or "jewel" varieties, and when I call for "sweet potatoes," I'm referring to the starchier, yellower vegetable. They can be used interchangeably, though I'm specific in this cookbook because of the differences in color.

Salt Preferences

I confess I use very little salt in my recipes, but that is mainly because I eat mostly whole foods, not sodium-laden processed ones, so my desire for salt has decreased substantially over the years. People tend to oversalt their food, and when making a recipe, it's the most difficult thing to reverse. I recommend salting at the very end of cooking, or just keep it low and let people salt their own portions. Either way, I indicate "salt, to taste" in many recipes, because I want you to find the level that works for you.

The Usual Suspects

As in *The Vegan Table*, each recipe in *Color Me Vegan* indicates whether it is oil-, wheat-, or soy-free, the first being a concern for people eating an oil-free diet and the latter two being common allergens. Recipes that need advance planning are indicated by the note "advance preparation required." As far as butter, I think Earth Balance is the only nondairy butter worth recommending. It is available in soy-free, organic, whipped, and baking sticks and can be used in every way that dairy-based butter is used.

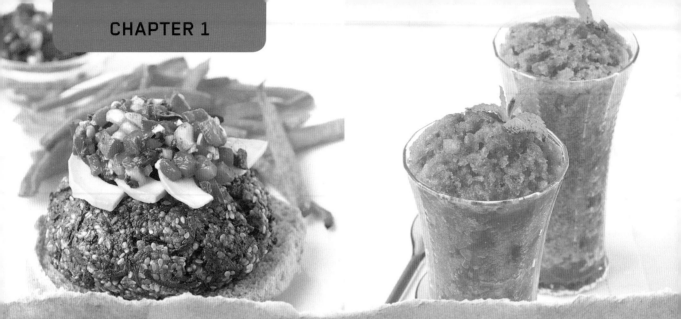

color me
ReD

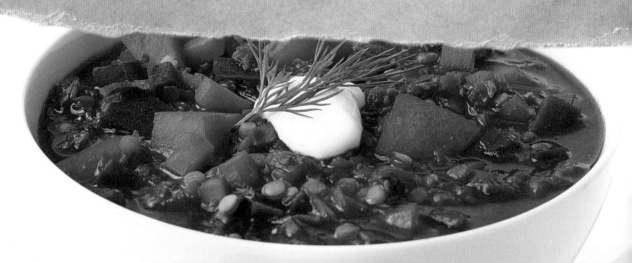

Although **anthocyanins** are the most dominant pigments in blue, purple, and deep red foods, a few other phytochemical pigments are at work, too.

Loopy for Lycopene

Lycopene (a type of carotenoid) and betacyanins are pigments most associated with tomatoes and beets, respectively. Lycopene is the pigment responsible for making tomatoes red and watermelon, grapefruit, guava, and papaya pink. Lycopene concentrates itself in certain organs of the body, primarily the lungs and the prostate gland. A number of studies show promising results in terms of lycopene's ability to prevent and treat prostate cancer, heart disease, breast cancer, macular degeneration, cataracts, and many other conditions.

Cook and Add Fat to Increase Absorption

It's not just a matter of consuming the nutrients we need but also a matter of increasing our absorption of them. The best way to increase the absorption of lycopene is to eat lycopene-rich vegetables *cooked*. Cooking frees the pigment that is tightly bound to the cell walls and makes it available for our bodies to use. This does not mean that you should abandon eating raw tomatoes! It means that including a combination of cooked and raw tomatoes and tomato-based foods will increase your body's ability to use lycopene. It also does not mean you should get your lycopene from ketchup. While lycopene is found in ketchup, most of the things people eat with ketchup aren't exactly on my list of "health food"—namely burgers and fries. However, if you switch out deep-fried french fries for baked carrot or yam fries (like the Carrot Fries on page 59), then dip away! Because lycopene is fat-soluble, another way to increase absorption is to prepare it with a little fat, which helps transport it to the bloodstream. Do this by making some tomato sauce with a small amount of olive oil, sautéing tomatoes with olives, eating tomatoes with avocado, and making the Roasted Plum Tomatoes with Garlic on page 29. Even when it comes to watermelon, you can eat it with some nuts or seeds or brush a little oil on it and grill it with other fruit.

Beneficial Betacyanins

Betacyanins also play a dominant role in the red color of certain plants like beets, red carrots, red grape skin, red chard, elderberry, and red cabbage. Preliminary research indicates their protective powers, particularly in the field of cancer.

Red Recipes

Enjoy recipes featuring beets, cherries, cranberries, red peppers, strawberries, tomatoes, watermelon, red chard, red lentils, and red miso. Other healthful red plant foods not necessarily featured but available at a market near you include red quinoa, red okra, rhubarb, pomegranate seeds, and chokecherries. Open your eyes—and your mouth—to the vast world of red-hued foods.

Apple, Cranberry, Cherry, and Pomegranate Salad

▶ *Oil-free, soy-free if using soy-free yogurt, wheat-free*

This simple and light dessert, snack, or breakfast is a winner not only for its flavor but also for its varied textures: chewy, creamy, crunchy, and crispy. It's also a powerful combination of four incredibly healthful red fruits: apples, cherries, cranberries, and pomegranate seeds.

4 red-skinned apples, chopped (not peeled)
¼ cup (27 g) blanched slivered almonds, toasted
¼ cup (40 g) chopped dried cherries or ½ cup (78 g) pitted and halved fresh cherries
¼ cup (27 g) dried cranberries
¼ cup (44 g) chopped dates
1 cup (245 g) nondairy vanilla yogurt
1 tablespoon (15 ml) lemon juice (optional)
¼ cup (27 g) pomegranate seeds

DIRECTIONS

In a medium bowl, combine the apples, almonds, cherries, cranberries, dates, yogurt, and lemon juice until all the ingredients are thoroughly combined.

Divide the salad among 4 plates and sprinkle each with the pomegranate seeds. This salad will hold up well in the fridge overnight, especially if you add the lemon juice to act as a natural preservative.

YIELD: 4 servings

SERVING SUGGESTIONS AND VARIATIONS

- Use toasted pecans, walnuts, or hazelnuts instead of almonds.
- Offset the sweetness of the dried fruit by using tart apples.
- Instead of vanilla yogurt, try other flavors, such as lemon or blueberry.

PER SERVING: 236 Calories; 5g Fat (18.4% calories from fat); 4g Protein; 48g Carbohydrate; 6g Dietary Fiber; 0mg Cholesterol; 9mg Sodium

did you know?

Quercetin is a powerful antioxidant found in the skins of apples (and red onions). Boasting anti-inflammatory, antihistamine, and anticancer properties, quercetin should be consumed through food, not supplements.

Roasted Red Pepper Relish

▶ *Wheat-free, soy-free*

A quick-to-prepare appetizer for an unexpected guest or a great side dish for burgers or wraps, this is a beautiful dish to show off.

2 roasted red peppers (fresh or from a jar), finely chopped
½ cup (50 g) finely chopped kalamata olives
2 cloves garlic, pressed or crushed
1 shallot, finely chopped
1 tablespoon (15 ml) balsamic vinegar
1 tablespoon (15 ml) olive oil
2 tablespoons (5 g) chopped fresh basil
1 tablespoon (5 g) chopped fresh parsley
Salt and freshly ground pepper, to taste

DIRECTIONS

Combine all the ingredients in a large bowl. Store for a week in the refrigerator or serve right away. The longer it keeps, the more the flavors will intensify.

Serve on toasted baguette slices or grilled polenta squares.

YIELD: 1½ to 2 cups (375 to 500 g)

PER SERVING: 20 Calories; 2g Fat (69.8% calories from fat); trace Protein; 1g Carbohydrate; trace Dietary Fiber; 0mg Cholesterol; 47mg Sodium

compassionate cooks' tip

The finely chopped roasted red peppers should yield ½ to ¾ cup (90 to 135 g).

food lore

The word *relish* comes from the Old French word *reles* (or *relais*), meaning "scent, taste, aftertaste" or more poetically, "a flavor that is left behind; a taste that lingers." Because of the presence of the vinegar, olives, and garlic, the flavor does indeed linger.

Cherry Tomatoes Stuffed with Green Olive Tapenade

▶ *Wheat-free, soy-free*

A world of flavor in each bite, this gorgeous recipe is courtesy of friends Barry and Jennifer Jones-Horton. Barry, who served for several years as head chef at the award-winning Ravens Restaurant of the Stanford Inn in Mendocino, California, now runs Local Love, a vegan organic food services company, with his wife Jennifer in Oakland, California.

20 cherry tomatoes
1 cup (100 g) pitted green olives
1 tablespoon (9 g) capers
1 clove garlic, minced
1 to 2 tablespoons (15 to 30 ml) lemon juice
2 tablespoons (30 ml) olive oil
Chopped parsley, for garnish
Lemon zest, for garnish

DIRECTIONS

Cut the top off each cherry tomato and, using a melon baller or a sharp knife, carefully scoop out the seeds and pulp. Place each tomato shell upside down on paper towels to drain.

Meanwhile, place the olives, capers, garlic, lemon juice, and olive oil in a blender or food processor and blend until smooth.

Divide the tapenade among each tomato cavity, sprinkle with parsley and lemon zest, and serve right away or place in the refrigerator for at least an hour to let the flavors mingle.

YIELD: 20 servings

PER SERVING: 22 Calories; 2g Fat (75.0% calories from fat); trace Protein; 1g Carbohydrate; trace Dietary Fiber; 0mg Cholesterol; 55mg Sodium

compassionate cooks' tips

• I make a distinction between oil-free and fat-free cooking and eating. In the early 1990s, we were bombarded with news stories about the healthfulness of oil, inspired primarily by the popularity of the Mediterranean Diet. It is not so much *oil* that is healthful but rather the healthful fats of whole foods, such as olives. I encourage people to eat plant fats in their whole state through nuts, seeds, olives, and avocados. This tapenade is an example of a healthful whole fat derived from the olives. Oil should be a small percentage of a healthful whole foods diet.

• The amount of tapenade you use depends on the size of your tomatoes. If you have some extra, spread it on some little toasts.

food lore

Green and black olives are not actually different types of olives. The difference is that green olives are picked from the tree before they're ripe, and black olives are left to ripen on the tree until they turn black. This is why black olives are softer in texture and less bitter than green olives.

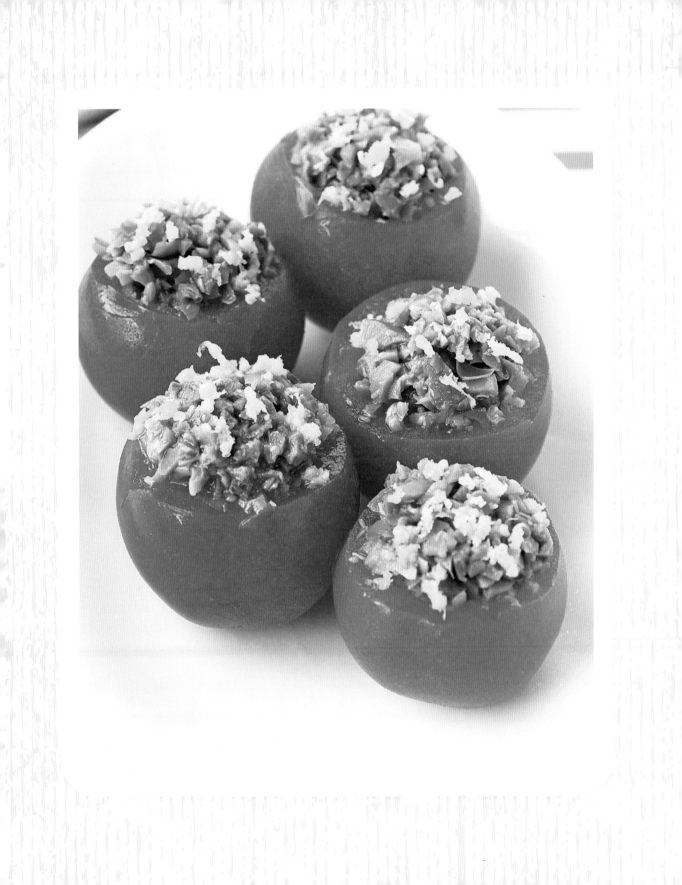

HOW ANTIOXIDANTS WORK

We often hear that antioxidants are a good thing, but we don't necessarily understand why. To understand the benefits of antioxidation, we first have to comprehend the effects of oxidation. It's a phenomenon we witness every time we cut into an apple or potato and the flesh begins to brown or when bicycle spokes turn rusty or a copper penny turns green. Oxidation occurs in everything from living tissues to base metals.

In short, oxidation occurs when oxygen interacts with a vulnerable surface (such as exposed fruit flesh). It's not always a bad thing, but it can be destructive. For instance, free radicals promote beneficial oxidation that produces energy and kills bacterial invaders. However, in excess, free radicals produce harmful oxidation that can damage cells. *Antioxidants*, such as those found in plant foods, fight free radicals and prevent them from causing damage.

The degenerative diseases we're grappling with today, such as cancer, cataracts, arthritis, and heart disease, to name but a few, are in many ways caused by oxidative damage. The research being done on phytochemicals, particularly those with antioxidant properties, suggests that the more antioxidants we consume (i.e., through fruits and vegetables), the more we increase our chances of repairing the damaged cells and thus preventing and treating certain diseases.

Antioxidant Recommendations

Although there is still much research to be done on the benefits of antioxidants, two things are certain: they are best obtained from food (not pills), and there is no upper limit for consuming them through food. Because antioxidants as a group aren't considered nutrients, except when they're vitamins or minerals, there are no specific recommendations for daily requirements. Although there are troublesome findings in research conducted on antioxidant *supplements* (see pages 86 and 87), experts agree that there is no upper intake level for antioxidants in *food*.

In other words, it is not recommended that people take vitamin E supplements (in addition to the small amount of vitamin E found in most multivitamins), but it is recommended that people take in vitamin E through food. It is not recommended that people take beta-carotene supplements, but it is recommended that people take in beta-carotene (which the body converts into vitamin A) through food.

So pile on the fruits and veggies and begin reaping the benefits—in both taste and health!

advance preparation required

Gazpacho

▶ *Soy-free, oil-free, wheat-free*

A chilled tomato soup originating in Spain, gazpacho is a refreshing soup in the hot-weather months and is often called a "liquid salad." Some versions feature chopped veggies, some feature minced, and some are puréed completely. This recipe incorporates a little of each method.

4 large or 6 medium ripe, red tomatoes, quartered

1 cucumber, peeled and coarsely chopped

½ red onion, coarsely chopped

3 cloves garlic, peeled

¼ cup (60 ml) water or fresh tomato juice, plus more if needed

2 tablespoons (30 ml) fresh lemon juice

2 tablespoons (30 ml) red wine, sherry, or apple cider vinegar

2 teaspoons (2 g) finely chopped fresh basil

1 tablespoon (13 g) granulated sugar

1 teaspoon (5 g) salt, or to taste

Freshly ground pepper, to taste

¼ cup (10 g) chopped fresh parsley

1 avocado, chopped

3 scallions, chopped

DIRECTIONS

To a food processor or blender, add the tomatoes, cucumber, red onion, garlic cloves, water or tomato juice, lemon juice, vinegar, basil, sugar, and salt. Purée until smooth or pulse if you prefer it to be slightly chunky. Add additional water or tomato juice to find the thickness you prefer.

Refrigerate for at least 2 hours or overnight.

When ready to serve, season to taste with salt and pepper and garnish with fresh parsley, chopped avocado, and chopped scallions.

YIELD: 4 servings

PER SERVING: 161 Calories; 8g Fat (42.1% calories from fat); 4g Protein; 22g Carbohydrate; 5g Dietary Fiber; 0mg Cholesterol; 568mg Sodium

food lore

The word *gazpacho* (which has no real English translation) has become a generic term for "cold soup." Other types of gazpacho can be made with avocados, cucumbers, watermelon, or grapes.

Six-Shades-of-Red Soup

▶ *Oil-free, wheat-free*

A rich-tasting and rich-colored soup, this recipe is a testament to how delicious low-calorie food can be.

10 cups (2350 ml) water

2 cups (400 g) red lentils, picked through and rinsed

3 red potatoes, unpeeled and chopped

2 red beets, peeled and diced

1 red onion, diced

2 carrots, finely chopped

2 cloves garlic, minced

½ teaspoon crushed red pepper flakes

1 tablespoon (2 g) finely chopped dill, plus more for garnish

¼ to ½ cup (65 to 130 g) red miso paste, depending on how strong it is

½ cup (120 ml) vegetable juice

1 teaspoon salt, or to taste

Freshly ground pepper, to taste

DIRECTIONS

Add the water, lentils, potatoes, beets, onion, garlic, red pepper flakes, and 1 tablespoon (2 g) dill to a large soup pot. Cover, bring to a boil, and then reduce the heat and simmer for 20 to 25 minutes or until the potatoes are fork-tender. (Keep covered while cooking.)

Meanwhile, in a small bowl, thoroughly combine the miso and juice. When the soup is done, remove from the heat, stir in the miso mixture, and serve topped with a sprinkling of fresh dill.

YIELD: 8 servings

SERVING SUGGESTIONS AND VARIATIONS

Purée half the soup and return to the pot for a thicker, creamier version.

PER SERVING: 263 Calories; 1g Fat (3.8% calories from fat); 16g Protein; 49g Carbohydrate; 11g Dietary Fiber; 0mg Cholesterol; 967mg Sodium

did you know?

There are more than 100 varieties of edible potatoes, ranging in size, shape, color, starch content, and flavor. They are classified as either "mature potatoes" (the larger ones most people are familiar with) or "new" potatoes (the smaller variety, which are harvested before maturity). Red potatoes are of the "new" variety and include Red LeSoda and Red Pontiac, both of which are nutritionally beneficial, particularly when consumed with their skins on!

compassionate cooks' tip

This soup, like so many, freezes well.

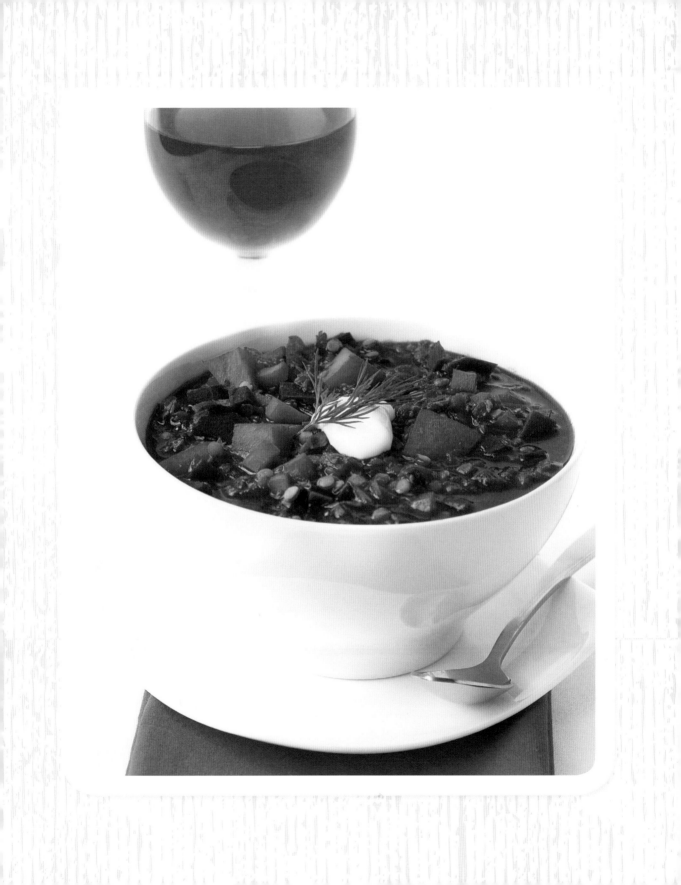

Apricot Red Lentil Stew

▶ *Soy-free, wheat-free, oil-free if sautéing in water*

The apricots add a touch of sweetness and cook down into melt-in-your-mouth goodness.

2 tablespoons (30 ml) oil or water, for sautéing

1 medium yellow onion, chopped

2 cloves garlic, minced

½ cup (88 g) halved dried apricots

1½ cups (300 g) red lentils, picked through and rinsed

5 cups (1175 ml) vegetable stock

3 Roma (plum) tomatoes, seeded and chopped

½ teaspoon ground cumin

½ teaspoon dried thyme

½ teaspoon salt, or to taste

Freshly ground black pepper, to taste

1 can (15 ounces, or 420 g) chickpeas, rinsed and drained

DIRECTIONS

Heat the oil in a large soup pot. Add the onion, garlic, and apricots and cook for about 7 minutes over medium heat until the onions begin to turn translucent. Stir occasionally to prevent sticking.

Add the lentils and stock. Cover, bring to a boil, and then reduce the heat and simmer for 30 minutes.

Stir in the tomatoes, cumin, thyme, and salt and pepper to taste. Simmer for 10 minutes.

Purée half of the stew in a blender or in a food processor (or use an immersion blender) and then return it to the pot. Add the chickpeas, cooking the stew until heated through, about 5 minutes. Serve hot.

YIELD: 4 to 6 servings

PER SERVING: 364 Calories; 7g Fat (15.7% calories from fat); 17g Protein; 62g Carbohydrate; 13g Dietary Fiber; 0mg Cholesterol; 1239mg Sodium

food lore

Leaving fruits out to dry in the sun and air is one of the oldest methods of preserving food. It enabled people to journey far with nutritious sustenance, preserve fruit for the winter, and add flavor and texture to savory dishes. There are many ways to use dried fruit in cooking:

• Add dried cranberries to a grain dish.

• Sprinkle raisins and dried berries on your morning cereal or oatmeal.

• Add sun-dried tomatoes to pasta dishes.

• Pair dried apricots with walnuts for muffins and breads.

• Mix dried cherries into granola or trail mix.

compassionate cooks' tip

If you would like to retain the chewy texture of the dried apricots, add them at a later stage in the cooking process.

Tomato Basil Soup

▶ *Soy-free if using soy-free Earth Balance, wheat-free*

Fresh basil and fresh tomatoes are the key to this simple and refreshing soup.

4 Roma or vine-ripe tomatoes, peeled, seeded, and diced
4 cups (940 ml) tomato juice
20 large fresh basil leaves
1 cup (235 ml) nondairy milk (such as almond, soy, rice, hazelnut, hemp, or oat)
3 tablespoons (42 g) nondairy butter (such as Earth Balance)
Salt and freshly ground pepper, to taste

compassionate cooks' tip

I've made this soup without peeling the tomatoes first, and even my high-powered blender can't guarantee a perfectly smooth soup, so if that's what you want, you'll need to peel the tomatoes first.

DIRECTIONS

Place the tomatoes and juice in a large soup pot over medium heat. Simmer for 30 minutes. Transfer the tomato mixture to a food processor or blender along with the basil leaves and purée until smooth. Return the purée to the soup pot.

Place the pot over medium heat and stir in the milk and butter. Season with salt and pepper. Heat, stirring, until the butter is melted but do not bring to a boil. Serve hot.

YIELD: 4 servings

HOW TO PEEL TOMATOES

1. Fill a saucepan three-quarters full of water, place over high heat, cover, and bring to a boil.
2. Place your tomatoes in the boiling water for 1 minute.
3. Using a slotted spoon, remove the tomatoes and set aside to cool.
4. Once they're cool enough to handle, gently pierce the skin of the tomatoes with the tip of a sharp knife. Loosen the skin with the knife and peel the skin away.

SERVING SUGGESTIONS AND VARIATIONS

- Some soups are even better the next day. This is one of them.
- If you're craving this soup in the winter, you may use canned peeled tomatoes.

PER SERVING: 133 Calories; 9g Fat (57.7% calories from fat); 4g Protein; 11g Carbohydrate; 4g Dietary Fiber; 0mg Cholesterol; 882mg Sodium

Harvard Beets

▶ *Wheat-free, soy-free if using soy-free Earth Balance*

Myths swirl around the origin of the name of this recipe. Supposedly created by a Harvard student, it is also reputed to have originated in a tavern in England named "Harwood," with "Harvard" being the mispronunciation of the name.

3 pounds (1365 g) fresh beets (about 5 medium), scrubbed clean
½ cup (120 ml) fresh orange juice
⅓ cup (67 g) granulated sugar
4 teaspoons (11 g) cornstarch
½ cup (120 ml) apple cider vinegar
2 tablespoons (28 g) nondairy butter (such as Earth Balance)
Salt, to taste
1 tablespoon (3 g) minced fresh parsley

compassionate cooks' tip

To roast the beets, preheat the oven to 400°F (200°C, or gas mark 6). Trim the greens from the beets (save the greens and sauté with garlic and olive oil), leaving at least 1 inch (2.5 cm) of the stems attached so the red pigment will not leak out during the cooking process. Place the unpeeled, whole beets in a large casserole dish, adding some water to the bottom of the dish and drizzling the beets with olive oil. Cover the casserole dish with foil and roast for about 1 hour and 15 minutes or until the beets are fork-tender. When they're cool enough to handle, slip the skin off, cut the stem off, and dice into bite-size chunks.

DIRECTIONS

There are many methods for cooking beets. For this recipe, you may quarter and steam them, remove the skins once they're cool enough to handle, and then dice them. Alternatively, you may boil them after quartering and peeling first and then dice them when they're cooked through. Finally, you may also roast them, outlined in the tip below.

While your beets are cooking by way of your preferred method, in a medium-size pot over medium heat, whisk together the orange juice, sugar, cornstarch, and vinegar. Make sure the cornstarch dissolves completely. Bring the mixture to a gentle boil, whisking constantly. Once it's thickened a bit, remove from the heat and stir in the butter until melted.

When the beets are cooked, peeled, and diced, stir them into the sauce. You may return the pot (with the beets) to the heat to serve them warm, or you can serve them at room temperature. Either way, add salt to taste and serve with minced parsley sprinkled on top. The contrast between the red and green is just gorgeous.

YIELD: 8 servings

SERVING SUGGESTIONS AND VARIATIONS

Choose from gold beets, red beets, and Chiogga beets.

PER SERVING: 120 Calories; 3g Fat (20.2% calories from fat); 2g Protein; 23g Carbohydrate; 3g Dietary Fiber; 0mg Cholesterol; 90mg Sodium

Roasted Plum Tomatoes with Garlic

▶ *Wheat-free, soy-free*

This is an incredibly easy recipe to prepare that can be served as a meal starter (as in a "roasted salad") or as a side dish. Fresh in-season tomatoes work best, but it is also a great way to use tomatoes that are starting to soften. I urge you to use fresh herbs for this—not dried!

8 Roma (plum) tomatoes, halved
12 cloves garlic, unpeeled
¼ cup (60 ml) olive oil
5 bay leaves
Salt and freshly ground pepper, to taste
3 tablespoons (8 g) finely chopped fresh oregano
2 tablespoons (5 g) finely chopped fresh basil
Rosemary sprigs, for garnish

did you know?

Tomatoes are packed with lycopene, a powerful antioxidant most closely associated with reduced risk of prostate cancer. However, though raw tomatoes are wonderful to eat for their flavor and nutrients, when it comes to lycopene, our bodies are better able to extract it when the tomatoes are cooked. And because lycopene is a fat-soluble phytonutrient, preparing cooked tomatoes with some oil also increases absorption.

DIRECTIONS

Preheat the oven to 450°F (230°C, or gas mark 8). Lightly oil an ovenproof dish into which the tomatoes fit snugly. Place the halved tomatoes in the dish (cut side up) and push the garlic cloves between them.

Brush the tomatoes with the olive oil, randomly stick the bay leaves in between the tomatoes, and sprinkle with salt and pepper.

Bake for 45 minutes or until the tomatoes have softened and charred around the edges. Sprinkle the oregano and basil all over the tomatoes and season with salt and pepper, if desired. Garnish with some rosemary sprigs for a pretty presentation.

YIELD: 4 servings

SERVING SUGGESTIONS AND VARIATIONS

If you can use a pretty ovenproof dish that you can transfer from oven to table, that would be ideal. This is truly an eye-catching—albeit simple—dish.

Toast some pine nuts and sprinkle on the finished recipe or just after you portion out individual servings.

PER SERVING: 188 Calories; 15g Fat (65.3% calories from fat); 3g Protein; 15g Carbohydrate; 3g Dietary Fiber; 0mg Cholesterol; 24mg Sodium

Apple, Cranberry, and Sausage Stuffing

▶ *Soy-free if using soy-free Earth Balance, wheat-free if using wheat-free bread*

This is a hearty, autumnal stuffing perfect for holiday feasts, meant to stuff your guests and not a bird.

5 cups (250 g) cubed bread of choice

1 tablespoon (15 ml) oil or (14 g) nondairy butter (such as Earth Balance)

1 pound (455 g) vegetarian sausage, coarsely chopped

1 large yellow onion, chopped

3 stalks celery, finely chopped

2 teaspoons dried sage

1 teaspoon dried rosemary

½ teaspoon dried thyme

½ teaspoon dried tarragon

1 tart apple, cored and chopped (not peeled)

¾ cup (90 g) dried cranberries

1 cup (100 g) pecans or walnuts

⅓ cup (20 g) minced fresh parsley

1½ cups (355 ml) vegetable stock

2 to 3 tablespoons (28 to 42 g) nondairy butter (such as Earth Balance), melted

DIRECTIONS

Preheat the oven to 350°F (180°C, or gas mark 4).

Spread the bread cubes in a single layer on a large baking sheet. Bake for 7 to 10 minutes or until evenly toasted. Transfer to a large bowl.

Meanwhile, in a large sauté pan, heat the oil and add the sausage, onion, and celery. Cook over medium-high heat for about 10 minutes, or until everything is evenly browned, stirring occasionally. Add the sage, rosemary, thyme, and tarragon to the sauté pan. Stir to combine.

Remove from the heat and add the sausage/onion mixture to the bread in the bowl. Stir in the chopped apple, dried cranberries, nuts, parsley, and vegetable stock, and mix thoroughly.

Transfer to a 9 x 13-inch (23 x 33 cm) casserole dish and drizzle with the melted butter. Bake for 30 to 40 minutes, stirring once, or until the top is golden brown.

YIELD: 8 to 10 servings

SERVING SUGGESTIONS AND VARIATIONS

- The best sausage for this would be Field Roast's Smoked Apple Sage Sausage, available in natural foods stores. Check out www.fieldroast.com. Other options include Tofurky sausage.
- Add more stock if you like it moister.

PER SERVING: 250 Calories; 15g Fat (52.5% calories from fat); 8g Protein; 22g Carbohydrate; 5g Dietary Fiber; 0mg Cholesterol; 511mg Sodium

WHY ARE SALMON PINK?

When we think of the color of salmon flesh, we tend to think *pink*. Or, to be more accurate, we tend to think of the color "salmon," which is a shade of pink that gets its name from this carnivorous fish. Salmon have been marketed as "health food," largely because of the omega-3 fatty acids their flesh contains, and some experts will even tout the health benefits derived from the pink color.

But just as the omega-3 fats in salmon are derived from the algae and algae-eating fish the salmon consume, so, too, do they get their characteristic pink-orange hue from aquatic plants—once removed.

As carnivores, salmon eat other animals, particularly zooplankton, herring, and krill. Krill, a small shrimp-like critter, eats phytoplankton (considered the "grass of the sea") as well as algae. Algae are made up of, among other things, omega-3 fats and carotenoids, the latter of which are responsible for turning krill *and* salmon pink. It is the algae that provide the nutritional benefit—not the fish.

Colorful Carotenoids

Powerful antioxidants, carotenoids, provide the red, orange, and yellow colors to various plants and play an important role in photosynthesis. The particular carotenoid pigment primarily responsible for turning salmon pink is called *astaxanthin*. Salmon and trout are unique in the way their muscles store it, which affects the color of their flesh.

Farmed Fish

With East Coast wild salmon all but extinct and West Coast wild salmon endangered, 90 percent of the salmon consumed in the United States is farm-raised in intensive confinement, replete with antibiotics and pesticides. Fed a diet of cheap fish meal made up of ground-up fish, farmed salmon do not consume their normal diet of crustaceans and thus range in color from gray to pale yellow. To appease consumers who have grown accustomed to pink-fleshed salmon (or "red-meat" rainbow trout), producers add to their feed *canthaxanthin*, a synthetic petrochemical-based dye manufactured by Hoffmann-La Roche, and other manufactured astaxanthins.

The point is that for human and many nonhuman animals, the nutrients we need are plant-based. The most concentrated source of omega-3 fatty acids is flaxseed, golden or brown. Buy them whole, grind them in a coffee grinder, and store them in the refrigerator or freezer once they're ground. Consume 1 tablespoon (7 g) ground flaxseed (or ground hemp seeds) each day in your salad, soup, oatmeal, cereal, or fruit smoothie.

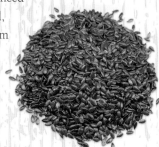

Quick Curried Swiss Chard

▶ *Wheat-free, soy-free*

I make this pretty frequently, because I always have these ingredients on hand.
It's a quick meal for dinner or to make in advance for lunch.

1 tablespoon (15 ml) coconut oil
1 large red onion, sliced
1 large bunch Swiss chard, chopped
1 teaspoon or more (to taste) curry paste
   (red or green)
1 cup (235 ml) nondairy milk (such as almond,
   soy, rice, hazelnut, hemp, or oat), divided
Salt, to taste

DIRECTIONS

Heat the coconut oil in a large sauté pan or wok over medium heat. Add the red onion, and cook for 5 to 7 minutes, stirring occasionally.

Add the chard and stir into the onion until they both begin to cook down and shrink in size.

Meanwhile, in a small bowl, stir the curry paste into a small amount of the 1 cup (235 ml) milk so that it becomes fully incorporated. Add it and the rest of the milk to the pan.

Stir the chard/onion mixture to combine it with the curry and milk and cook for 5 or 10 minutes, uncovered, to fully tenderize the chard and deepen the flavor of the curry. You don't want to cook it so long that the milk totally evaporates. It makes a delicious sauce over rice.

Add salt to taste and serve hot over brown rice or the Coconut Rice on page 176. It is also delicious served at room temperature.

YIELD: 2 servings

SERVING SUGGESTIONS AND VARIATIONS

If you don't have coconut oil, you may use olive; the coconut oil just increases the flavor of the dish.

PER SERVING: 136 Calories; 11g Fat (66.8% calories from fat); 4g Protein; 8g Carbohydrate; 3g Dietary Fiber; 0mg Cholesterol; 110mg Sodium

did you know?

Both the stalks (whether red, white, yellow, or orange) and the leaves of chard are edible, but because the stems tend to vary in texture, some may be more tender than others. Chard is packed with vitamins K, A, and C, along with vitamin E, fiber, folate, calcium, iron, and potassium.

compassionate cooks' tip

Red-stemmed Swiss chard makes this suitable for the red chapter, but any color chard will do.

Seared Tempeh with Cherry Balsamic Reduction Sauce

▶ *Wheat-free*

This is the perfect dish when cherries are in season in late spring. However, dried cherries will work just as well.

1 package (10 ounces, or 280 g) tempeh, cut into ½-inch (1.3 cm) strips

3 to 4 tablespoons (45 to 60 ml) olive oil, divided

2 tablespoons (30 ml) water

3 tablespoons (40 g) granulated sugar

1 cup (155 g) fresh halved cherries or ½ cup (60 g) dried cherries

3 tablespoons (45 ml) balsamic vinegar

1 yellow onion, sliced

4 cloves garlic, minced

1 cup (235 ml) dry red wine

½ cup (120 ml) vegetable stock

½ cup (120 ml) nondairy milk (such as almond, soy, rice, hazelnut, hemp, or oat)

DIRECTIONS

Steam the tempeh for 10 minutes in a steamer basket placed in a pot filled with a small amount of water. Tempeh can have a little bit of a bitter taste to it, and steaming takes the edge off. It also tenderizes it and increases absorption of whatever flavors you add to it.

Heat a large skillet with 2 tablespoons (30 ml) of the olive oil over medium-high heat and sear the tempeh until it's crispy on one side, about 5 minutes. Turn and do the same on the second side. Each side should be golden brown. Remove the tempeh from the skillet and set aside on a plate lined with paper towels (to absorb some of the oil).

In a small saucepan, combine the water and sugar and gently stir over medium-high heat until the sugar is completely dissolved. Immediately remove the pan from the heat and stir in the cherries and balsamic vinegar. (If the sugar hardens after you add the cherries and vinegar, just return the saucepan to low heat and gently stir until the sugar melts once more.) Remove the pan from the heat and set aside.

Meanwhile, in the skillet you used for the tempeh, heat the remaining 1 to 2 tablespoons (15 to 30 ml) olive oil, and add the onion and garlic. Sauté until the onion turns translucent, about 5 minutes.

Add the wine, bring the mixture to a boil, and boil until reduced to around ⅔ cup (155 ml).

Add the stock, return the mixture to a boil, and cook until reduced to ⅔ cup (155 ml) again.

Stir in the milk and the cherry mixture and cook for just 5 more minutes until it's reduced a little more and thickened up.

Divide the tempeh between 2 plates and top with the sauce.

YIELD: 2 servings

SERVING SUGGESTIONS AND VARIATIONS

Serve the tempeh and sauce over a bed of rice, on a mound of mashed potatoes, or on a bed of sautéed greens.

PER SERVING: 777 Calories; 40g Fat (48.8% calories from fat); 30g Protein; 64g Carbohydrate; 3g Dietary Fiber; 0mg Cholesterol; 349mg Sodium

Beet Burgers

▶ *Wheat-free if using quinoa or millet instead of bulgur*

I had been wanting to replicate a favorite beet burger from a local restaurant for a long time, and I'm totally tickled to have done so with this recipe. This burger pairs perfectly with a side of carrot fries (see page 59).

2 cups (240 g) grated beets (about 2 large beets)

1½ cups (300 g) cooked bulgur wheat (or quinoa or millet)

1 cup (130 g) toasted sunflower seeds

½ cup (120 g) toasted sesame seeds

½ cup (80 g) minced onion (about 1 small onion)

½ cup (60 g) bread crumbs

¼ cup (60 ml) oil

3 tablespoons (24 g) all-purpose flour

3 tablespoons (8 g) finely chopped fresh parsley

4 cloves, garlic finely chopped

2 to 3 tablespoons (30 to 45 ml) tamari soy sauce

¼ teaspoon cayenne pepper, or to taste

Salt, to taste

DIRECTIONS

Preheat the oven to 350°F (180°C, or gas mark 4). Line a baking sheet with unbleached parchment paper.

In a large bowl, combine the grated beets, bulgur, sunflower seeds, sesame seeds, onion, bread crumbs, oil, flour, parsley, garlic, tamari, and cayenne. Add salt to taste.

At this point, test if you can create a patty that will stay together. These are definitely softer-type burgers, but you should still be able to form a patty with no problem. If it still falls apart, add a little more bulgur or flour until you have a firm patty that won't fall apart while cooking/baking.

Continue forming uniform-size patties. I make mine a little bulky and get about 12 patties out of them. You can also make them a little smaller and less dense.

Bake for 25 minutes or until firm. Carefully flip halfway during the cooking time.

Serve each burger on a whole wheat bun, topped with sliced tomatoes, grilled red onions, avocado slices, and eggless mayonnaise. (Wildwood's Garlic Aioli and Follow Your Heart's Vegenaise are my favorites.)

YIELD: 10 to 12 patties

SERVING SUGGESTIONS AND VARIATIONS

Instead of baking, you can fry these with a little oil in a sauté pan.

PER SERVING: 225 Calories; 16g Fat (60.8% calories from fat); 6g Protein; 17g Carbohydrate; 5g Dietary Fiber; 0mg Cholesterol; 122mg Sodium

compassionate cooks' tip

These burgers freeze very well. To freeze, form the patties and place a piece of parchment between each one before storing in a freezer-safe container. Thaw before baking and flip halfway through the cooking.

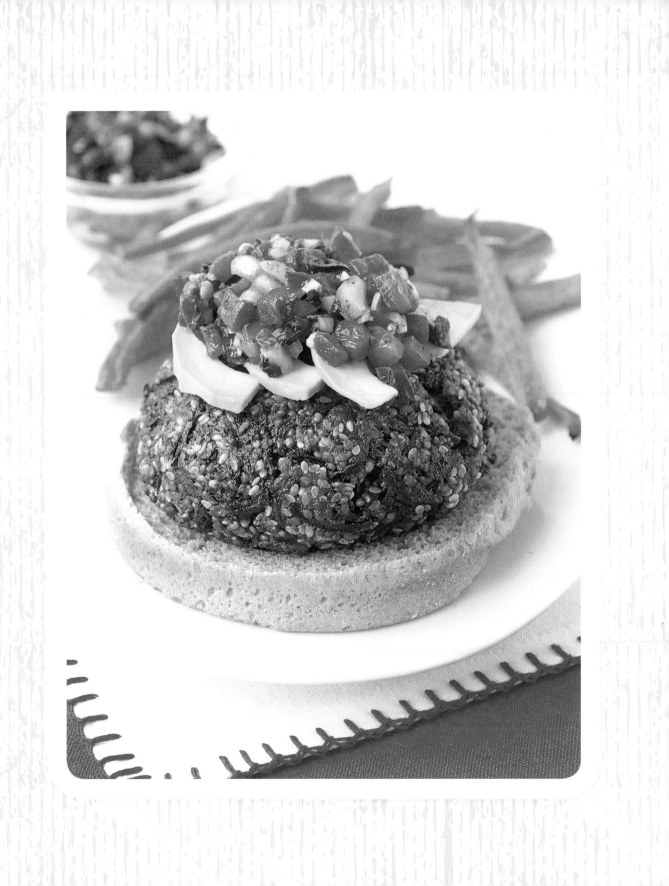

Stuffed Shells with Marinara Sauce

▶ *Oil-free*

Baked, the tofu ricotta has a wonderful creamy texture, which nicely complements the chewy pasta noodles and the spinach filling.

16 to 24 jumbo pasta shells

2 packages (10 ounces, or 280 g) frozen chopped spinach, thawed and drained

12 ounces (340 g) soft tofu

12 ounces (340 g) extra-firm tofu

1 tablespoon (13 g) granulated sugar

¼ cup (60 ml) nondairy milk (such as almond, rice, soy, hemp, hazelnut, or oat)

1 teaspoon garlic powder

1 teaspoon onion powder

2 tablespoons (30 ml) lemon juice

1 bunch fresh basil, minced

2 teaspoons (10 g) salt

4 to 6 cups (980 to 1470 g) tomato sauce, divided

2 teaspoons minced fresh parsley

2 teaspoons minced fresh thyme

2 teaspoons minced fresh oregano

3 tablespoons (27 g) toasted pine nuts, ground to a soft crumble

Salt and freshly ground pepper, to taste

DIRECTIONS

Preheat the oven to 350°F (180°C, or gas mark 4). Lightly oil a 9 x 13-inch (23 x 33 cm) baking dish. Cook the pasta shells according to package directions, drain well, and set aside. Squeeze the spinach as dry as possible and set aside.

Place the tofus, sugar, milk, garlic powder, onion powder, lemon juice, basil, and salt in a food processor or blender and blend until smooth. Transfer to a large bowl and stir in the spinach.

Stuff about 2 rounded tablespoonfuls (30 g) into each pasta shell. Spread 1 cup (245 g) or so of tomato sauce over the bottom of the prepared baking dish. Arrange the stuffed shells in a single layer over the sauce and spoon the remaining 3 to 5 cups (735 to 1225 g) sauce over the shells. Sprinkle with the fresh parsley, thyme, and oregano.

Bake until heated through, about 35 to 45 minutes. Sprinkle with the toasted pine nuts, additional fresh herbs, if desired, and salt and pepper, to taste.

YIELD: 8 servings

SERVING SUGGESTIONS AND VARIATIONS

Make a batch of garlic bread to serve with the shells. Mince several cloves of garlic and mix with a couple teaspoons of olive oil and paprika. Cut a baguette in half lengthwise and place on a baking sheet, face up. Spread the bread with the garlic mixture and bake in a 400°F (200°C, or gas mark 6) oven for 15 minutes or until the bread is crisp.

PER SERVING: 252 Calories; 6g Fat (21.2% calories from fat); 15g Protein; 38g Carbohydrate; 7g Dietary Fiber; 0mg Cholesterol; 1661mg Sodium

did you know?

The word *marinara* means "of the sea" but loosely translates as "sauce of the sailors." Originating in Naples, Italy, in the sixteenth century, marinara sauce was a meatless sauce used on sailing ships. Because it contained no animal products (which spoil) and because the high acid content of the tomatoes preserved the sauce, it was perfect for long voyages.

Cajun Red Beans and Rice

▶ *Wheat-free or soy-free, depending on the sausage used*

Stoke the fire on a cold winter's night and enjoy this hearty, flavorful stew-like dish.

1 tablespoon (15 ml) oil

2 cloves garlic, minced

1 medium onion, diced

1 green bell pepper, diced

4 links (about 12 ounces, or 340 g) vegetarian sausage, sliced into rounds and then halved

2 teaspoons "Cajun" or "Creole" seasoning

1 cup (185 g) uncooked long-grain brown rice

3 cups (705 ml) water

1 can (15 ounces, or 420 g) dark red kidney beans, drained and rinsed

2 tablespoons (8 g) minced fresh parsley

DIRECTIONS

Heat the oil in a soup pot over medium heat. Add the garlic, onion, and pepper and sauté until the vegetables are tender, about 7 minutes.

Add the sausage and brown a bit. Add a wee bit more oil, if necessary.

Stir in the Cajun seasoning and rice and toast for about a minute. Add the water, being sure to scrape up all the browned bits from the bottom of the pot, and the beans. Bring to a boil. Cover, reduce the heat to low, and cook until the rice is done, 35 to 40 minutes. Add the parsley and stir to combine.

Remove from the heat and let stand for a few minutes (with the lid still on). Serve hot.

YIELD: 4 servings

PER SERVING: 353 Calories; 7g Fat (18.2% calories from fat); 14g Protein; 60g Carbohydrate; 10g Dietary Fiber; 0mg Cholesterol; 640mg Sodium

compassionate cooks' tips

• Use Tofurky's or Field Roast's Italian Sausage. The former is tofu-based; the latter is wheat-based, and they're both delicious.

• To make your own "Cajun" or "Creole" seasoning, combine 2 tablespoons (11 g) cayenne pepper, 2 tablespoons (14 g) paprika, 1½ tablespoons (10 g) onion powder, 2 tablespoons (12 g) freshly ground black pepper, 1 tablespoon (9 g) garlic powder, 2 teaspoons dried basil, 1 teaspoon chili powder, ¼ teaspoon dried thyme, ¼ teaspoon ground mustard, ⅛ teaspoon ground cloves, and salt to taste.

advance preparation required

Watermelon Granita

▶ *Soy-free, oil-free, wheat-free*

Next to eating fresh watermelon, this is my favorite way of enjoying this juicy summer fruit. It's pretty, it's easy, and it contains lots of beta-carotene and lycopene.

⅓ cup (132 g) granulated sugar

⅓ cup (80 ml) water

4 cups (560 g) seedless watermelon chunks, reserving the wedges for garnish

Juice of 1 lime

Mint leaves, for garnish

DIRECTIONS

Make a simple syrup by heating the sugar and water in a pan over high heat and stirring until all the sugar has dissolved. Set aside and let cool.

Add the cooled sugar syrup, watermelon chunks, and lime juice to a blender. Purée until smooth.

Pour into a shallow, wide pan and freeze for 1 hour. Rake the mixture with a fork and freeze for another hour. Rake and freeze for 1 more hour. The whole process takes about 3 hours. Rake before serving. It may be held in the freezer for up to 2 days.

Serve in margarita glasses or in large wine goblets to show off the color of the watermelon and the sparkle of the ice crystals. Garnish with the watermelon wedges and mint leaves.

YIELD: 4 servings

SERVING SUGGESTIONS AND VARIATIONS

- Granita, which translates simply to "ice," is so easy to make and incredibly versatile. Choose any liquid—pomegranate juice, champagne, even carrot juice—add some sugar and whatever other flavorings seem desirable, and stick it in the freezer. Rake with a fork every now and then, and you've got granita!
- Use yellow watermelon to make a yellow variety and serve yellow and red in different glasses for a very pretty effect.

PER SERVING: 154 Calories; trace Fat (1.8% calories from fat); 1g Protein; 39g Carbohydrate; trace Dietary Fiber; 0mg Cholesterol; 3mg Sodium

food lore

Related to sorbet and Italian ice, granita hails from Sicily and dates back to Arab rule in the region, when snow dealers would haul blocks of snow down from Mount Etna. Depending on the location, the texture of granita range from granular and icy to slushy.

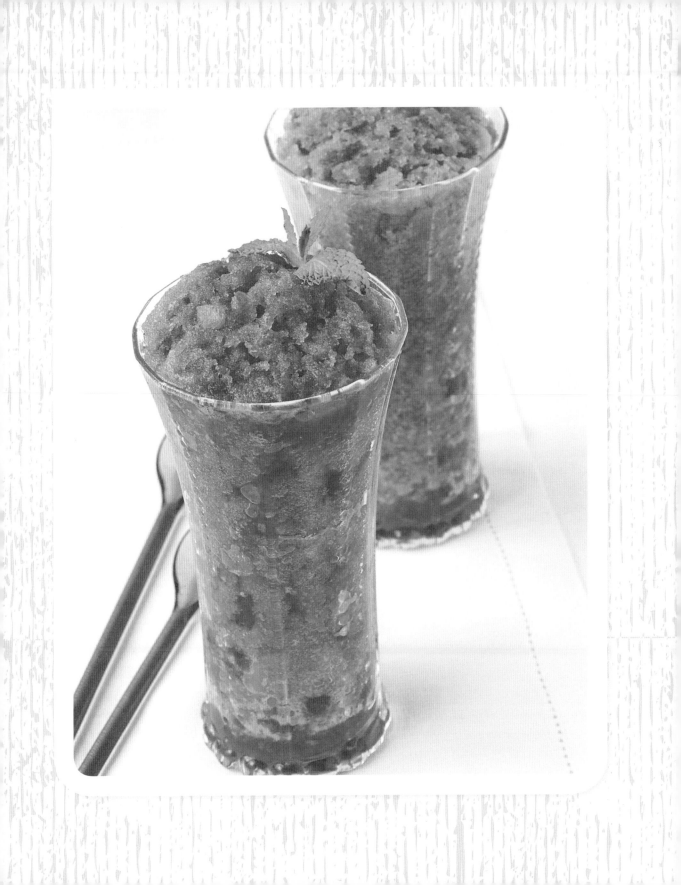

Strawberry Lemonade

▶ *Soy-free, oil-free, wheat-free*

This refreshing and gorgeous drink is hugely popular at summertime soirees.

7 ice cubes

1 cup (235 ml) fresh lemon juice
(about 6 medium lemons)

5 cups (1175 ml) cold water

1 cup (200 g) granulated sugar (more or less,
depending on your sweet preference)

6 to 8 whole strawberries, stems removed, plus
6 strawberries for garnish

DIRECTIONS

I like to crush the ice a little first, so I add the ice cubes to my blender and pulse a few times until they're broken up a bit. Next, add the lemon juice, water, and sugar. Blend until smooth and taste. You may like it sweeter and will want to add more sugar, you may like it more tart and will want to add more lemon juice, or you may want to just dilute it with more water. Find the level that works for you.

Next, add the whole strawberries. My preference is to leave the strawberries somewhat chunky, so I do not purée it until smooth. I pulse a few times to break up the strawberries into pieces. The result is not only very pretty, but it's also very satisfying to catch strawberry pieces in your mouth with each sip!

Serve cold in individual glasses with a whole strawberry on the rim or add to a pitcher.

YIELD: 6 servings

SERVING SUGGESTIONS AND VARIATIONS

• After juicing the lemons, I quarter what's remaining of them (the skin and rind) and throw them into the pitcher.

• Make Strawberry Limeade, using limes instead of lemons.

• Never one to resist providing several options, I have to pass on what one of my testers suggested as an adult variation once the sun goes down: add a little vodka and serve in a pretty martini glass with a lemon wedge.

PER SERVING: 144 Calories; trace Fat (0.3% calories from fat); trace Protein; 38g Carbohydrate; 1g Dietary Fiber; 0mg Cholesterol; 1393mg Sodium

compassionate cooks' tips

• For those who have a food processor (see Recommendations), use the juicer attachment to juice the lemons in no time.

• If you don't have a food processor, juice the lemons using a manual juicer (they're very convenient) or do them by hand. Roll them first between your hand and countertop before cutting in half and juicing. It loosens them up a bit.

Raspberry Lemon Muffins

▶ *Soy-free, if using soy-free yogurt and milk*

These delicious little muffins are satisfying any time of the day.

1 container (6 ounces, or 170 g) vanilla or plain nondairy yogurt

½ cup (120 ml) nondairy milk (such as almond, soy, rice, hazelnut, hemp, or oat)

3 tablespoons (45 ml) canola oil

Juice from 1 lemon (about 2 tablespoons)

½ teaspoon lemon extract (optional)

1½ cups (180 g) all-purpose or whole wheat pastry flour

¾ cup (150 g) granulated sugar

2½ teaspoons (12 g) baking powder

¼ teaspoon salt

1 teaspoon lemon zest

1 cup (125 g) fresh raspberries, or (250 g) frozen

DIRECTIONS

Preheat the oven to 400°F (200°C, or gas mark 6). Lightly grease a 12-cup muffin tin or line with cupcake liners (paper or silicone).

In a large bowl, mix together the yogurt, milk, oil, lemon juice, and lemon extract.

In a separate bowl, stir together the flour, sugar, baking powder, salt, and lemon zest. Add the wet ingredients to the dry and mix until just blended. Gently fold in the raspberries.

Spoon the batter evenly into the prepared muffin cups.

Bake for 20 to 25 minutes or until the top springs back when lightly touched. Cool the muffins in the tin on a wire rack.

YIELD: 12 muffins

SERVING SUGGESTIONS AND VARIATIONS

• Use fruit yogurt instead of plain or vanilla.
• Replace the raspberries with blueberries, peaches, or cherries—frozen or fresh.

PER SERVING: 154 Calories; 4g Fat (23.4% calories from fat); 2g Protein; 28g Carbohydrate; 1g Dietary Fiber; 0mg Cholesterol; 109mg Sodium

compassionate cooks' tips

• In any recipe that calls for lemon zest and lemon juice, it's a good idea to zest the lemon before juicing the lemon.

• I have had great success with the silicone cupcake liners. They reduce a little fat and calories (because you don't have to grease the muffin tin), and they make cleanup a breeze. I use them whenever I make cupcakes or muffins.

Strawberry Cream

▶ *Wheat-free, oil-free*

This is a simple, versatile, decadent cream perfect as a topping for fruit, pound cake, or dessert waffles.

2 containers (8 ounces, or 225 g) nondairy
  cream cheese, at room temperature
  (Tofutti is a good brand)
½ cup (115 g) nondairy sour cream
½ cup (50 g) confectioners' sugar
¾ cup (185 g) puréed fresh strawberries
  (10 large strawberries)

DIRECTIONS

In a food processor, process the cream cheese until smooth. Add the sour cream, sugar, and strawberries. Process until smooth and creamy, scraping down the sides of the bowl as needed. Refrigerate for up to 1 week.

YIELD: 2 cups (800 g)

SERVING SUGGESTIONS AND VARIATIONS

Use as a filling for a layered cake, strawberry short-cake, or éclairs.

PER SERVING: 92 Calories; 2g Fat (12.6% calories from fat); 3g Protein; 30g Carbohydrate; 4g Dietary Fiber; 0mg Cholesterol; 9mg Sodium

compassionate cooks' tip

Tofutti brand makes a great sour cream, but you can also make your own by puréeing silken tofu with a souring agent, such as lemon juice.

WAYS TO INCREASE RED FOODS

- Add red bell peppers to your salad or stir-fry.

- Add red or pink rose petals to a salad or sprinkle them over a sweet dessert.

- Drink tomato juice. (Try and find a low-sodium version.)

- Eat red watermelon or make juice from fresh watermelon.

- Roast, boil, or steam beats and make a beet salad.

- Shred raw beets onto a green salad.

- Add raw beets to your juicer, along with some carrots, ginger, and apples for a delicious juice.

- Keep a store of tomato sauce for making quick pizzas or pasta dishes.

- Eat salsa with tortilla chips.

- Add pomegranate seeds to a leafy green or citrus salad.

- Drink pomegranate juice.

- Eat raspberries as a snack or add them to a salad or smoothie.

- Make a tomato salad (quarter a red tomato, sprinkle on some salt and freshly ground pepper, and drizzle on a little olive oil).

- Add dried cherries to your oatmeal or salad.

- Add frozen cherries to your breakfast smoothie or make a cherry crumble.

- Choose red grapefruit for a snack or breakfast.

- Add sun-dried tomatoes to salads, sautés, and pasta.

- Roast red peppers.

- Make your own trail mix with dried cherries.

- Drink cranberry juice (find a low-sugar version).

- Eat raw red bell peppers with hummus.

- Add tomato paste to soups and stir-fries.

- Snack on unpeeled red-skinned apples.

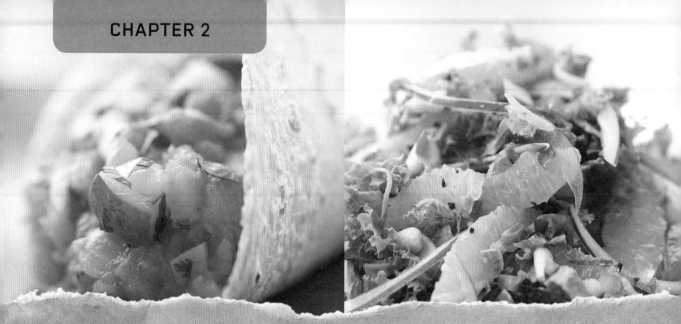

color me

oraNGe

THE "BETA" TO SEE YOU WITH

Although beta-carotene usually receives the most attention, it is only one of about 600 similar compounds called *carotenoids* that are present in many fruits and vegetables (including carrots, from whence they get their name). Aside from beta-carotene, the five other major carotenoids include *alpha-carotene, lycopene, beta-cryptoxanthin, lutein,* and *zeaxanthin.* High carotenoid intake has been linked with decreased risk for postmenopausal breast cancer and for cancers of the bladder, cervix, prostate, colon, larynx, and esophagus.

Gray Areas in Color Boundaries

The color of carotenoids can range from pale yellow to bright orange to deep red, so I could just as easily introduce the carotenoid family in the yellow chapter as in the red or orange—or more significantly, in the green (see page 102). However, the average person tends to be more familiar with beta-carotene than with any of the other carotenoids. Beta-carotene is, in fact, what contributes to the orange color of many different fruits and vegetables, such as sweet potatoes and cantaloupe melon. Generally, the greater the intensity of the orange color of the fruit or vegetable, the more beta-carotene it contains.

Alpha Before Beta

Leaving aside our common friend beta-carotene, it's worth familiarizing ourselves with another carotenoid, alpha-carotene. Like beta-carotene, it also converts into vitamin A in our bodies and plays an important role in the health of our eyes. And it appears that it may be an even stronger antioxidant than beta-carotene, so stay tuned! (Antioxidants are essentially enzymes that stop free radicals from causing cells to break down, or *oxidize*, and cause damage that can lead to such diseases as heart disease and cancer.)

Fat-Solubility

Keep in mind that just because we're *eating* these protective substances, it doesn't necessarily mean we're *absorbing* them. Carotenoids are fat-soluble, so eating them with some fat increases the absorption through the digestive tract. The Carrot and Avocado Salad on page 228 is a perfect way to take in some good fat along with a carotenoid-rich food, as is the Carrot Purée (page 56) atop the Roasted Fennel (page 178).

You Can't Always Judge a Carotenoid by Its Color

Although oranges are, well, orange, it is not because of beta-carotene. The carotenoids beta-cryptoxanthin, zeaxanthin, and lutein are dominant in these yummy fruits. So, without beta-carotene to convert into vitamin A, it is safe to say that citrus fruits like oranges are not a great source of this vitamin. They are, however, and an excellent source of vitamin C and folate and help our bodies absorb iron. As far as citrus fruits go, only pink grapefruit boasts beta-carotene.

Citrus Salad

▶ *Soy-free, wheat-free, oil-free*

Enjoy this fresh, light, delicious salad any time of the year.

1 bunch curly kale, leaves stripped from rib and finely chopped

2 oranges, peeled with membranes removed and separated into wedges

1 red grapefruit, peeled with membranes removed and separated into wedges

1 small red onion, thinly sliced

1 jalapeño pepper, seeded and minced, or ⅛ teaspoon crushed red pepper flakes

2 tablespoons (18 g) toasted pine nuts

¼ cup (60 ml) fresh orange juice

Juice from 1 lime

1 tablespoon (15 ml) vinegar (apple cider, balsamic, or rice)

2 tablespoons (40 g) agave nectar (or other liquid sweetener)

Zest from 1 orange, for garnish

DIRECTIONS

Add the kale, oranges, grapefruit, onion, jalapeño pepper, and pine nuts to a large bowl and set aside.

In a separate bowl, whisk together the orange juice, lime juice, vinegar, and agave nectar. Pour the mixture over the salad ingredients and toss gently to coat evenly.

Serve in individual bowls, garnished with orange zest.

YIELD: 4 servings

SERVING SUGGESTIONS AND VARIATIONS

Any type of kale works well for this salad, though curly is my favorite.

PER SERVING: 137 Calories; 2g Fat (12.6% calories from fat); 3g Protein; 30g Carbohydrate; 4g Dietary Fiber; 0mg Cholesterol; 9mg Sodium

compassionate cooks' tip

To "supreme" a citrus fruit means to remove the skin, pith, membranes, and seeds and separate into wedges, as requested in the ingredients list. To accomplish this, cut a thin slice off the top and bottom of each fruit (orange, tangerine, grapefruit), exposing the flesh. Stand each orange upright and cut off the peel, removing all of the white pith and membrane as you cut. If the peel was especially thick, you may end up with a slightly misshapen fruit. Now cut the exposed orange into segments or wedges.

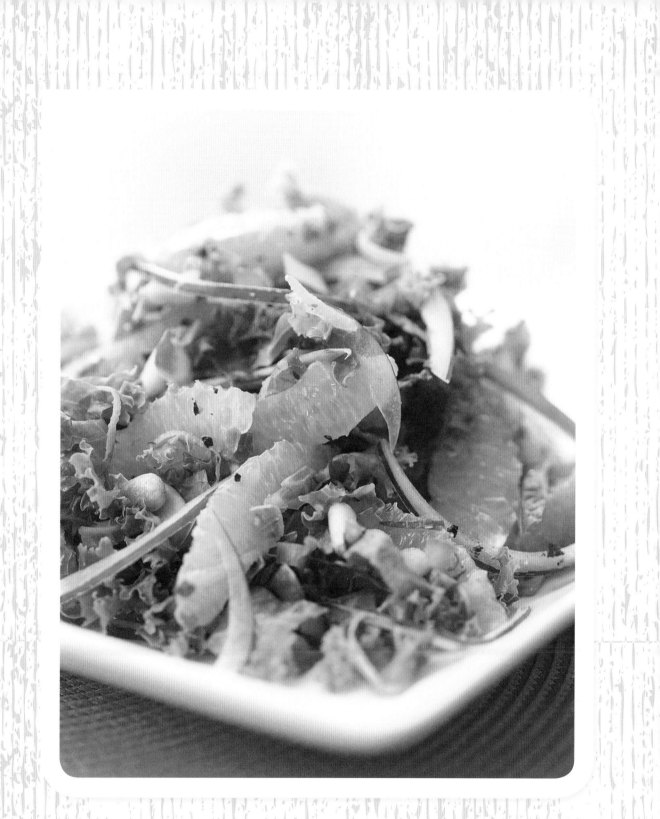

Orange Pecans

▶ *Wheat-free, soy-free if using soy-free Earth Balance*

Flavored nuts are a wonderful treat to put out for party guests or just to snack on throughout the day.

2 tablespoons (28 g) nondairy butter
  (such as Earth Balance)
4 teaspoons (16 g) grated orange zest
  (from about 2 large oranges)
2 teaspoons ground cinnamon
1 teaspoon ground coriander
½ teaspoon ground cloves
¼ teaspoon cayenne pepper
2 cups (200 g) raw pecan halves
2 tablespoons (26 g) granulated sugar
1 teaspoon salt
Zest from 1 orange, for garnish

DIRECTIONS

Preheat the oven to 300°F (150°C, or gas mark 2). Line a baking sheet with parchment paper.

Melt the butter in medium saucepan over low heat. Add the orange zest, cinnamon, coriander, cloves, and cayenne pepper. Stir until aromatic, about 30 seconds.

Add the pecans, sugar, and salt and stir to coat evenly. Transfer the mixture to the baking sheet. Bake until the nuts are toasted, stirring occasionally, about 17 minutes and up to 20 minutes. Cool, and serve with additional zest sprinkled on top.

Store in an airtight container for up to a week.

YIELD: 8 servings, about ¼ cup (28 g) each

PER SERVING: 237 Calories; 22g Fat (80.0% calories from fat); 2g Protein; 10g Carbohydrate; 3g Dietary Fiber; 0mg Cholesterol; 306mg Sodium

compassionate cooks' tip

The nuts continue cooking a bit after you take them out of the oven, and they crisp up once they're cooled. Do not cook in the oven longer than 20 minutes or they will burn.

Roasted Orange Beets with Tangerines

▶ *Wheat-free, soy-free*

Earthy beets pair so well with citrus. As with many of the veggies that have more than one color to choose from, red beets can be used instead of orange, adding a striking contrast with the tangerines.

24 baby or 6 large orange beets

Olive oil, for drizzling

½ cup (120 ml) fresh orange juice

¼ cup (60 ml) olive oil

3 tablespoons (45 ml) raspberry vinegar

4 small shallots, thinly sliced

Salt and freshly ground pepper, to taste

8 tangerines, peeled with membranes removed and separated into segments

2 tablespoons (18 g) toasted pine nuts

compassionate cooks' tip

Tf you'd like to make part of this dish in advance, you may store the roasted beets in the refrigerator overnight. Bring to room temperature before proceeding with the recipe.

DIRECTIONS

Preheat the oven to 400°F (200°C, or gas mark 6).

Trim the greens from the beets (save the greens and sauté with garlic and olive oil), leaving at least 1 inch (2.5 cm) of the stems attached.

Place the unpeeled, whole beets in a large casserole dish, adding a little water to the bottom of the dish and drizzling the beets with olive oil. (You're kind of steam-roasting them; don't add so much water that the beets are swimming in it but add enough that the bottom of the dish doesn't burn.)

Cover the casserole dish with foil (you can even give the beets a little poke with a fork first) and roast for about 1 hour and 15 minutes or until the beets are fork-tender (less time for smaller beets, so check halfway through the cooking time). When they're cool enough to handle, slip the skin off, cut the stem off, and quarter the beets.

In a medium bowl, combine the orange juice, oil, raspberry vinegar, sliced shallots, and a pinch of salt and pepper. Whisk together until combined and set aside.

Arrange the quartered beets and tangerine sections on individual plates and drizzle with the dressing. Alternatively, marinate the beets in the dressing for about a half hour before serving as directed. Top with the toasted pine nuts and serve.

YIELD: 4 to 6 servings

PER SERVING: 277 Calories; 10g Fat (84.6% calories from fat); trace Protein; 4g Carbohydrate; 11g Dietary Fiber; 0mg Cholesterol; 313mg Sodium

Peach or Nectarine Salsa

▶ *Oil-free, wheat-free, soy-free*

The colors in this dish will knock your socks off, and the flavor will have your taste buds tingling for more. Fresh, light, and packed with nutrients, this salsa can be served as a topping, dip, or filling.

3 large ripe peaches or nectarines,
  cubed and unpeeled
1 red bell pepper, finely diced
½ red onion, finely chopped
2 tablespoons (30 ml) orange, lime,
  pineapple, or lemon juice
2 tablespoons (12 g) chopped fresh mint
1 tablespoon (9 g) finely chopped jalapeño
  or chipotle pepper
¼ teaspoon salt
1 teaspoon grated fresh ginger
2 tablespoons (30 ml) balsamic vinegar
1 teaspoon light brown sugar

DIRECTIONS
Combine all the ingredients in a large bowl and let sit for at least 5 minutes before tasting to adjust seasonings. Serve right away or chill in the fridge for a minimum of 1 hour or a maximum of 2 days.

YIELD: 32 servings, about 2 tablespoons (14 g) each

SERVING SUGGESTIONS AND VARIATIONS
• Serve with crackers or crispy corn chips.
• Serve as a topping on grilled tempeh, tofu, or mushrooms.
• Serve in burritos, fajitas, and countless other wrap-type foods.

PER SERVING: 7 Calories; trace Fat (2.8% calories from fat); trace Protein; 2g Carbohydrate; trace Dietary Fiber; 0mg Cholesterol; 17mg Sodium

did you know?

Peaches and nectarines are both stone fruits with similar taste and texture profiles, though nutritionally, nectarines pack a little more punch (with twice the amount of vitamin A, slightly more vitamin C, and much more potassium). The other main difference is that peaches have fuzzy skin and nectarines have smooth skin, but this slight difference makes discerners of us all. (I prefer nectarines.) Either way, leave the skin on to reap the maximum nutritional benefits.

compassionate cooks' tip

Because white peaches lack beta-carotene and vitamin A, choose yellow peaches for a healthier option.

Carrot and Roasted Bell Pepper Soup

▶ Oil-free, wheat-free

This is a delicious and beautiful soup good for any time of the year. Reduce the spicy cayenne, if you prefer, but its presence gives this soup a little kick!

3 carrots, peeled and chopped

2 yellow onions, coarsely chopped

1 yellow potato, peeled and coarsely chopped

3 cloves garlic, finely chopped

½ cup (120 ml) dry sherry or dry white wine (or nonalcoholic white wine)

¼ teaspoon salt, plus more to taste

2 roasted bell peppers (roast your own or use jarred), coarsely chopped

2 teaspoons fresh or 1 teaspoon dried thyme

3 cups (705 ml) vegetable stock

⅓ cup (83 g) yellow/light miso

2 cups (470 ml) nondairy milk (such as almond, soy, rice, hazelnut, hemp, or oat), divided

¼ teaspoon cayenne pepper

DIRECTIONS

In a soup pot, combine the carrots, onions, potato, garlic, sherry, and salt. Cook over medium heat until the liquid evaporates, about 10 minutes.

Add the roasted peppers, thyme, and stock. Cover and simmer until the carrots and potatoes are tender, about 25 minutes.

Transfer to a blender, working in batches if your blender is on the smaller side. Add the miso and 1 cup (235 ml) of the nondairy milk. Blend until smooth.

Return to the pot and slowly stir in the remaining 1 cup (235 ml) milk to achieve the desired thickness. Add the cayenne and more salt to taste. Reheat and serve.

YIELD: 4 to 6 servings

PER SERVING: 141 Calories; 3g Fat (20.6% calories from fat); 6g Protein; 22g Carbohydrate; 5g Dietary Fiber; 0mg Cholesterol; 1116mg Sodium

compassionate cooks' tip

Most jarred roasted peppers are of the red variety; to increase the orange color of this soup, roast your own orange bell peppers.

Butternut Squash Orange Ginger Soup

▶ *Wheat-free, soy-free, oil-free*

A delightfully sweet soup, it's as healing as it is delicious.

1 tablespoon (15 ml) water, for sautéing

1 large yellow or white onion, coarsely chopped

3 tablespoons (18 g) minced fresh ginger

4 cloves garlic, minced

¼ cup (60 ml) orange juice

1 large butternut squash, peeled, seeded, and cubed

2 medium yellow potatoes, peeled and quartered

3½ cups (823 ml) vegetable stock

Salt and freshly ground pepper, to taste

2 tablespoons (8 g) finely chopped fresh parsley or cilantro, for garnish

Zest from 2 oranges (about 2 tablespoons [6 g]), for garnish

2 scallions, thinly sliced or finely chopped, for garnish

DIRECTIONS

Add the water to a large soup pot over medium heat. Sauté the onion, ginger, and garlic for 5 minutes.

Add the orange juice, and simmer for about 3 minutes. Add the butternut squash, potatoes, and stock. Simmer slowly for about 25 minutes or until the squash and potatoes are fork-tender.

Ladle the contents into a blender and purée or use an immersion blender directly in the pot.

Return the puréed soup to the soup pot and reheat over low heat. Season with salt and freshly ground pepper, to taste, and divide among 4 to 6 bowls.

Garnish the individual servings with parsley, orange zest, and scallions and serve.

YIELD: 4 to 6 servings

PER SERVING: 197 Calories; 1g Fat (3.9% calories from fat); 4g Protein; 48g Carbohydrate; 6g Dietary Fiber; 0mg Cholesterol; 594mg Sodium

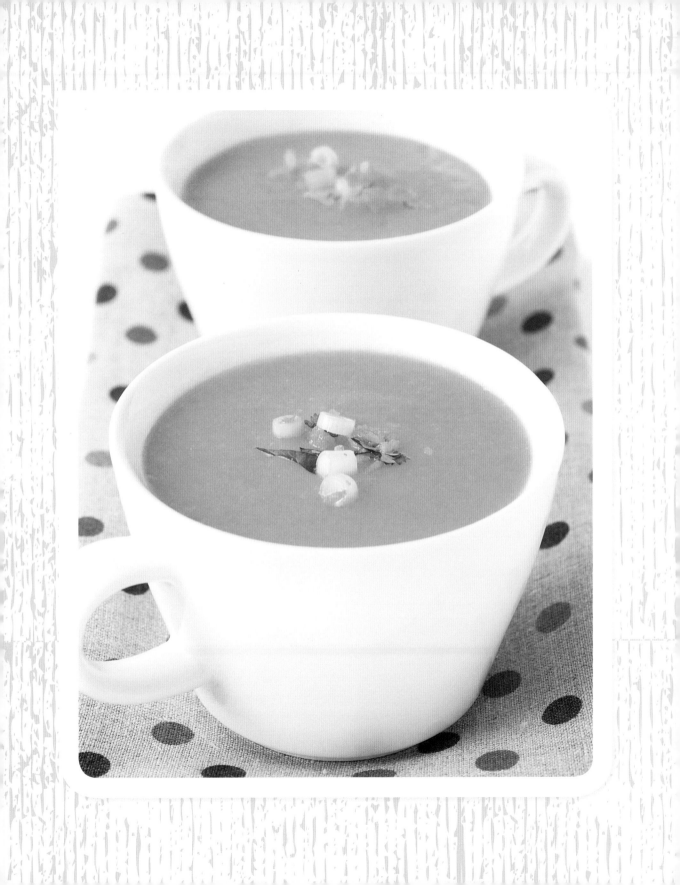

Peanut Pumpkin Soup

▶ *Wheat-free, soy-free, oil-free if using water to sauté*

Chock full of autumnal goodness, this is a filling and delicious hearty stew, attributed to Roger Hallsten, with whom I taught my very first cooking class many moons ago.

1 to 2 tablespoons (15 to 30 ml) water or oil, for sautéing

1 medium yellow onion, chopped

3 stalks celery, chopped

3 carrots, chopped

1 can (15 ounces, or 420 g) white beans (cannellini, Great Northern, or navy)

1 cup (235 ml) boiling or very hot water

½ to ¾ cup (130 to 195 g) smooth peanut butter

1 can (15 ounces, or 420 g) pumpkin purée (or the purée from 1 pumpkin to equal 1½ cups [338 g])

2 tablespoons (30 ml) white wine vinegar or white wine

2 dried bay leaves

1 teaspoon dried sage

1 teaspoon dried thyme

½ teaspoon (or more) crushed red pepper flakes

3 yellow potatoes, cubed but not peeled

4 cups (940 ml) water or vegetable stock

Salt, to taste

½ cup (73 g) peanuts, chopped

¼ cup (15 g) chopped fresh parsley

DIRECTIONS

Heat the water in a large soup pot. Add the onion, celery, and carrots. Sauté for 5 to 7 minutes or until the onions turn translucent.

Meanwhile, blend the boiling water with the peanut butter until smooth. Add it to the sautéed veggies along with the pumpkin purée, vinegar, bay leaves, sage, thyme, red pepper flakes, potatoes, and 4 cups (940 ml) water.

Lower the heat and simmer for 30 minutes or until the potatoes are fork-tender. For crunchier "al dente" carrots, you can add them in the last 5 minutes of cooking.

Remove the bay leaves, add salt to taste, and serve hot in individual bowls. Top with the ground peanuts and parsley.

YIELD: 4 servings

PER SERVING: 696 Calories; 36g Fat (43.2% calories from fat); 29g Protein; 76g Carbohydrate; 17g Dietary Fiber; 0mg Cholesterol; 1283mg Sodium

compassionate cooks' tip

If using whole pumpkins rather than canned, look for those called "sweet pumpkins" or pie pumpkins, which will be sweeter and less stringy than those used to carve jack-o'-lanterns.

did you know?

After carrots and yams, pumpkins contain more beta-carotene than any other food we eat. They also contain fair amounts of alpha-carotene, lutein, and zeaxanthin, all of which are associated with cancer prevention and tumor reduction.

Baked Persimmon Slices

▶ *Wheat-free, soy-free and oil-free if eliminating butter*

A very simple "recipe," this is one of my favorite ways to eat Fuyu persimmons (aside from eating them raw as a snack or adding them to salads).

4 Fuyu persimmons
1 to 2 tablespoons (14 to 28 g) nondairy butter
    (such as Earth Balance, optional), melted
Ground cinnamon

did you know?

Fuyu persimmons are crisp like an apple when ripe. Their skin—just like the skin of an apple—is absolutely edible and delicious. Look for deep orange skin when choosing. The Hachiya persimmon isn't really eaten until it's perfectly soft and ripe. The skin, more like that of a tomato, is usually discarded, while the flesh is usually puréed and often used in baked goods (see Persimmon Tea Cake on page 69).

food lore

The word *persimmon* means "dry fruit," reflecting its use by the Blackfoot, Cree, and Mohican tribes of the eastern United States.

DIRECTIONS

Preheat the oven to 350°F (180°C, or gas mark 4). Line a baking sheet with unbleached parchment paper.

Slice the persimmons as thinly as possible. Although you can slice them any way you like, their center star pattern is quite pretty, so I recommend slicing them crosswise to keep the pattern intact.

Brush a thin layer of nondairy butter on each slice, arrange the persimmons on the baking sheet in a single layer, and lightly sprinkle the top with cinnamon. If you prefer to keep the dish fat-free, skip the butter, still sprinkle with cinnamon, and continue as directed.

Bake for 10 minutes or until the ends start to curl up. Flip the persimmons over (they'll be moist on the underside) and bake for another 5 minutes, adding a wee bit more cinnamon, if desired. Allow to cool slightly before serving.

YIELD: 24 to 28 slices

SERVING SUGGESTIONS AND VARIATIONS

For dried persimmons, bake in a 100° to 130°F oven (40° to 55°C) for 24 hours or in a food dehydrator for 10 hours, or until dried and chewy.

PER SERVING: 12 Calories; 1g Fat (54.7% calories from fat); trace Protein; 1g Carbohydrate; trace Dietary Fiber; 0mg Cholesterol; trace Sodium

Carrot Purée

▶ *Wheat-free, oil-free, soy-free if using soy-free milk and Earth Balance*

This is a strikingly beautiful dish. I recommend serving this with something green, which will complement the bright orange of the purée.

½ cup (120 ml) vegetable stock
5 to 6 large carrots, cut into uniform chunks
½ teaspoon salt, plus more to taste
⅛ teaspoon ground cloves
1 to 2 tablespoons (15 to 30 ml) nondairy
    milk (such as almond, soy, rice, hazelnut,
    hemp, or oat)
1 tablespoon (15 g) light brown sugar or (20 g)
    maple syrup
1 tablespoon (14 g) nondairy butter (such
    as Earth Balance)

DIRECTIONS

Bring the stock to a boil. Add the carrots and salt. Cover and cook until soft, about 20 minutes, adjusting the heat to maintain a slow simmer. Drain the carrots (save the broth) and transfer to a food processor along with the ground cloves. Add the broth and milk (enough to get the consistency you want) and purée until almost smooth.

Add the brown sugar and butter and continue puréeing. Add more salt to taste.

Either serve as is or check out the serving suggestions below.

YIELD: 4 to 6 servings, about ⅓ cup (75 g) each

SERVING SUGGESTION AND VARIATIONS

• Bake in a lightly oiled baking dish for about 30 minutes until hot and bubbly.
• Serve as you would mashed potatoes—as a side dish—or add dollops of the purée (or pipe it using a pastry bag) onto roasted fennel slices and serve as a delectable appetizer. (See the Roasted Fennel recipe, page 178.)

PER SERVING: 60 Calories; 2g Fat (29.6% calories from fat); trace Protein; 10g Carbohydrate; 2g Dietary Fiber; 0mg Cholesterol; 289mg Sodium

did you know?

Carrots were originally red, yellow, and purple—not orange. In fact, no one had seen an orange carrot until they were bred in the Netherlands in the seventeenth century. For an unknown reason, orange carrots became the norm, though other color varieties are still available, like the purple-skinned and orange-fleshed ones we grow in our garden at home.

compassionate cooks' tip

Tempting though it might be, please forgo using so-called "baby carrots." They are bred to be small, not flavorful.

CRAZY FOR CARROTS

Because I love so many plant foods, I would be hard-pressed to pick a favorite. If the criterion, however, were the frequency with which I eat a particular plant food, then carrots would win. I eat a lot of carrots—raw, cooked, shredded, diced, julienned, and juiced.

Until the Dutch began breeding orange carrots in the seventeenth century, carrots were largely purple, yellow, or white. The jury is still out as to why they starting breeding them orange. As a result, however, carrots are very high in beta-carotene (the precursor to vitamin A) and also contain vitamin C, vitamin K, vitamin B6, folate, potassium, magnesium, other vitamins and minerals, and lots of dietary fiber. Although I eat primarily orange carrots, in my backyard garden, we also grow purple, red, white, and black varieties.

Baby Carrots

The only kind of carrots I don't eat are baby carrots. Now, before you curse me for blaspheming a seemingly perfectly innocent food, allow me to explain: I don't like them. I don't think they taste good. They lack the skin of real carrots. They lack the earthy flavor of real carrots. They are more expensive than real carrots. I just don't like them. There. I said it. Baby carrots aren't bred for their flavor, necessarily. They're bred to be sweeter, yes, but they're also bred to be consistently orange and small. They're bred to grow faster and ripen more quickly, and thus have only 70 percent of the beta-carotene of a normal carrot. So, I'm sticking with my story. I don't like baby carrots.

The Eyes Have It

One of the reasons beta-carotene is so significant is because our bodies convert it into vitamin A, which is important for maintaining and strengthening the immune system; keeping the skin, lungs, and intestinal track working properly; and promoting healthy cell growth. Vitamin A is also crucial for eyesight, so much so that its chemical name refers to the in our eyes.

Vitamin A is also found in a variety of dark green and deep orange, red, and yellow fruits and vegetables, such as sweet potatoes, pumpkin, spinach, butternut squash, turnip greens, bok choy, mustard greens, and romaine lettuce.

Taste and See

The elements that impart color (pigments) aren't the only reason for the protective nature of carrots; the compounds that impart also play a role. Terpineol, a phytochemical that enables carrots to fight off fungi and our bodies to fight off cancer, is responsible for the earthy flavor of carrots. Apigenin is another phytochemical—particularly a flavonoid—that boasts antioxidant, anti-inflammatory, and antitumor properties.

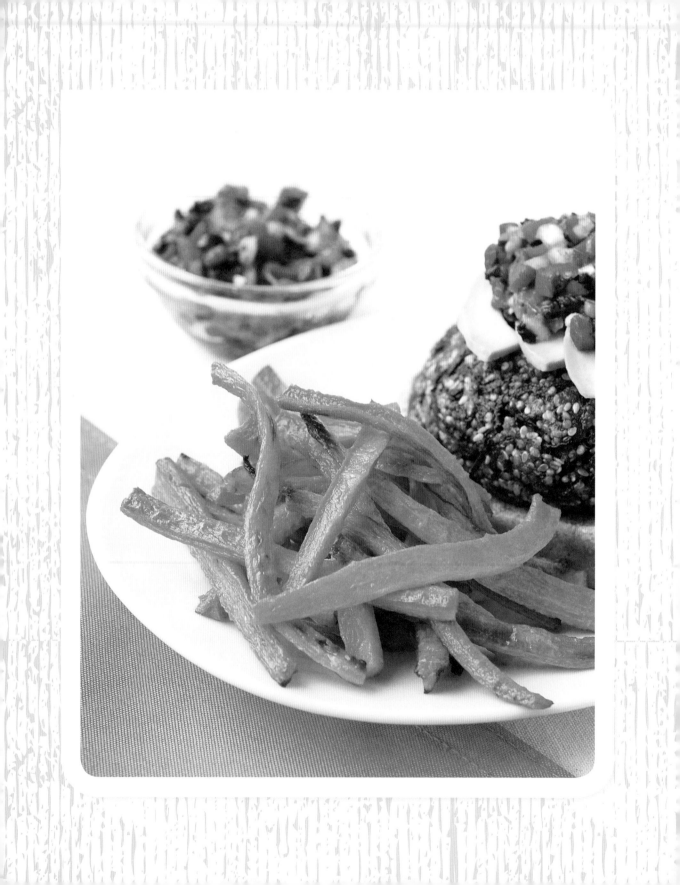

Carrot Fries

▶ *Soy-free, wheat-free*

Mega amounts of beta-carotene result in these gorgeous-color fries that pack a nutritional as well as flavorful punch. Cooked just right, they yield a combination of crispy and satisfyingly chewy results.

16 medium carrots, peeled and cut into
    matchsticks about 4 inches (10 cm) long
1 tablespoon (15 ml) oil
1 teaspoon salt
Freshly ground pepper, to taste
½ teaspoon ground cumin (optional)

did you know?

When you eat a large amount of beta-carotene-rich foods, you may notice your skin begin to take on an orange glow. There is nothing wrong with this. However, if you want to tone down the tint, you can still eat carotenoid-rich foods that aren't orange. (To put it in perspective: one medium carrot contains 330 percent of your Daily Value of vitamin A; 1 cup [30 g] of raw spinach contains 75 percent.)

DIRECTIONS

Preheat the oven to 425°F (220°C, or gas mark 7).

Place the carrot sticks in a bowl and pour the olive oil over them. Using your hands, toss the carrots in the oil to thoroughly coat.

Spread the carrot sticks in a single layer on a baking sheet lined with parchment paper. Sprinkle with the salt, pepper, and cumin.

Bake the carrots until they begin to crisp, about 45 minutes, checking every 15 minutes or so to toss or turn the pan to ensure even cooking.

YIELD: 4 servings

SERVING SUGGESTIONS AND VARIATIONS

- When tossing the carrots with the oil, add a tablespoon of agave nectar and/or chili powder.
- Serve with the Blueberry Ketchup on page 145.
- These go great with Beet Burgers on page 34.

PER SERVING: 155 Calories; 4g Fat (21.9% calories from fat); 3g Protein; 29g Carbohydrate; 9g Dietary Fiber; 0mg Cholesterol; 634mg Sodium

Saffron Rice with Curried Apricot Dressing

▶ *Wheat-free, soy-free*

This recipe, adapted from San Francisco's Millennium Restaurant's cookbook, has been in my repertoire for years. Personalize it by adding your favorite root vegetables, such as carrots, sweet potatoes, turnips, and rutabagas.

1 tablespoon (15 ml) water or vegetable stock, for sautéing

1 medium yellow onion, finely diced

2 cloves garlic, minced

1 teaspoon ground cumin

1 teaspoon fennel seed

¼ teaspoon freshly ground pepper

½ teaspoon salt, or to taste

2 cups (380 g) uncooked brown basmati rice

½ teaspoon saffron steeped in ¼ cup (60 ml) warm water

3½ cups (823 ml) water or vegetable stock

2 cups (220 g) cubed garnet or jewel yams, steamed and cooled

1 tart apple, diced and tossed with lemon juice

3 scallions, thinly sliced

½ cup (68 g) toasted pine nuts

CURRIED APRICOT DRESSING

¼ cup (75 g) apricot preserves

⅓ cup (80 ml) rice vinegar

1 tablespoon (9 g) curry powder

¼ teaspoon ground cardamom

¼ teaspoon cayenne pepper

⅓ cup (80 ml) water

¼ cup (60 ml) oil

Salt, to taste

2 tablespoons (12 g) finely shredded mint leaves, for garnish

DIRECTIONS

In a medium saucepan, heat the water or stock over medium heat and sauté the onion and garlic until just softened, about 5 minutes. Add the cumin, fennel seed, pepper, and salt. Sauté for 1 minute. Add the rice and stir constantly for 2 minutes or until the rice smells fragrant. Add the saffron in the water as well as the 3½ cups (823 ml) water, bring to boil, and cover. Reduce the heat to low and simmer for 40 to 45 minutes or until the liquid is absorbed. Remove from the heat and transfer to a large bowl. To the bowl, add the yams, apple, scallions, and pine nuts. Set aside.

To make the dressing, combine all the ingredients in a blender or food processor and blend until emulsified. Taste and adjust the seasonings. Combine most of the dressing with the rice/veggie mixture and mix thoroughly. Taste and add the rest of the dressing, if desired, or reserve for another use. Arrange on a serving platter. Garnish with the mint.

YIELD: 6 to 8 servings

SERVING SUGGESTIONS AND VARIATIONS

- The dressing may be made in advance and kept in the refrigerator for up to a week.
- Served with a salad and bread (I imagine Indian or Middle Eastern breads, such as naan, roti, pita, or other flat breads), this dish is a meal in itself.

PER SERVING: 347 Calories; 13g Fat (31.2% calories from fat); 6g Protein; 57g Carbohydrate; 5g Dietary Fiber; 0mg Cholesterol; 586mg Sodium

Orange-Glazed Tempeh

▶ *Wheat-free*

Tempeh tends to be an unfamiliar food to most Westerners (it's a staple in Indonesia), though everyone enjoys it once they try it. It has a satisfying bite, a nutty flavor, and a versatile texture.

1 package (10 ounces, or 280 g) tempeh
2 tablespoons (30 ml) oil
1 cup (235 ml) freshly squeezed orange juice
   (from 3 or 4 oranges)
1 tablespoon (8 g) freshly grated ginger
2 tablespoons (30 ml) tamari soy sauce
1 tablespoon (15 ml) mirin or rice wine vinegar
1 tablespoon (20 g) real maple syrup
½ teaspoon ground coriander
3 cloves garlic, minced
Juice from ½ lime (optional)

compassionate cooks' tips

- By steaming the tempeh first, you tenderize this delicious soy-based food and eliminate some of the bitterness. Slice and steam for 10 minutes and cook as directed.

- Tofu may be used in place of tempeh.

- A microplane is a handy tool that grates ginger and zests lemons like nobody's business. Find it online or in kitchen supply stores.

DIRECTIONS

Cut the tempeh into slices that are not too thick (tempeh plumps up when it cooks) but not too thin. Heat the oil in a large sauté pan over medium heat and fry the tempeh until the slices are golden brown on one side. If your oil is hot enough, this should take only about 5 minutes. Turn the slices over and cook on the other side, adding a little more oil if necessary.

Meanwhile, in a medium bowl, combine the orange juice, fresh ginger, tamari, mirin, maple syrup, and coriander and stir to combine.

Once the tempeh is nice and crispy on both sides, pour the marinade into the pan, along with the garlic. Simmer for about 10 minutes or until the sauce has reduced to a thick glaze. Turn the tempeh once more during this time.

Serve the tempeh drizzled with any remaining sauce and a squeeze of lime. Serve over sautéed kale.

YIELD: 2 servings

SERVING SUGGESTIONS AND VARIATIONS

Serve with Peach or Nectarine Salsa (page 50).

PER SERVING: 526 Calories; 25g Fat (41.0% calories from fat); 29g Protein; 53g Carbohydrate; 1g Dietary Fiber; 0mg Cholesterol; 307mg Sodium

Sweet Potato Tacos (*Tacos de Papa*)

▶ *Wheat-free if using corn tortillas, soy-free*

During a weeklong stay at a magical eco-resort in Mexico called Majahuitas, we were treated to three glorious meals a day. Among our favorites were the potato tacos, which I've modified here to include orange sweet potatoes (a.k.a. yams). Yellow potatoes may be used instead.

2 large sweet potatoes (or yams), peeled and cubed
1 tablespoon (15 ml) olive oil
1 medium yellow onion, sliced
1 red or yellow bell pepper, finely diced
Salt and freshly ground pepper, to taste
2 cloves garlic, minced or pressed
¼ teaspoon cayenne pepper
½ fresh jalapeño pepper, seeded and diced
8 to 10 small crispy corn or soft flour tortillas
Chopped cilantro, for garnish
Salsa, for topping

DIRECTIONS

Place a steamer basket in a medium saucepan with enough water on the bottom of the pot to create steam. Place the cubed potatoes in the basket, cover, and steam over medium-low heat until fork-tender, about 20 to 25 minutes, and then drain. Be sure to keep an eye on the pot to ensure that your water doesn't evaporate, creating a burned saucepan.

Meanwhile, in a medium sauté pan over medium heat, heat the olive oil. Add the onion and diced bell pepper and cook for about 7 minutes or until the vegetables are translucent. Season with salt and pepper and set aside.

When the sweet potatoes are finished cooking, transfer them to a large bowl, along with the garlic, cayenne, jalapeño, pepper and onion mixture; add salt to taste. Mash all the ingredients together as you would mashed potatoes or leave somewhat chunky.

Fill the tortillas with the filling, sprinkle with chopped cilantro, top with peach salsa (see page 50), and serve. This makes a beautiful presentation!

YIELD: 8 to 10 servings

PER SERVING: 282 Calories; 7g Fat (21.2% calories from fat); 7g Protein; 48g Carbohydrate; 3g Dietary Fiber; 0mg Cholesterol; 348mg Sodium

compassionate cooks' tip

Because there is confusion about what constitutes a sweet potato and what constitutes a yam, I want to be clear. For this recipe, you may use the white or yellow starchier sweet potato or the creamier yam (either a garnet or a jewel). Depending on where you're from, they each have different names, but in this case, they can be used interchangeably.

food lore

We tend to associate potatoes with Ireland, so you may think "potato tacos" are a clash of cultures, but not if you consider that potatoes originated in Peru.

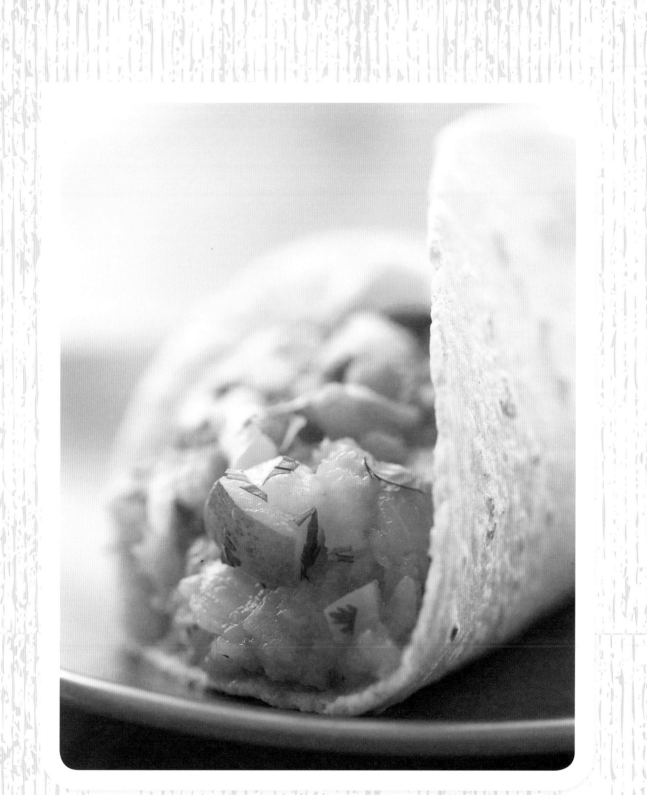

HOW TO CHOP ONIONS WITHOUT CRYING

I confess I never, ever cry while chopping onions. Ever. Not even so much as a small tear. Is it because I know the secret? Is it because I'm immune, as some experts suggest happens when you're around onions long enough? To be honest, I'm not really sure.

Why do onions make us cry in the first place? Well, as I discuss on page 163, onions contain a volatile sulfur gas called allicin, whose antibacterial effects deter *us* as much as they deter *bacteria*. When we chop an onion, we break apart cells that emit these gases that turn into sulfuric acid in the air, as vapor. To wash the irritating acid away, our eyes well up with tears. And the more we chop, the more we cry.

There are as many suggestions for preventing this as there are tears that form when we chop. Because I've never had this issue, I cannot attest to one working more than another, but here are some of the methods:

- Peel onions under running water to wash away the irritant.
- Wear swimming goggles to protect your eyes.
- Chop in a well-ventilated room, or buy a small fan to aim toward you while you chop.
- Chop quickly.
- Chop only chilled onions.
- Use a good, sharp chef's knife. It glides through the onion with ease, emitting fewer of the compounds that cause tears to come out.
- Put a slice of bread in your mouth, with half of it sticking out to "catch" the fumes.
- Burn a candle or turn on the gas burner immediately adjacent to where you're chopping. The tear-causing gas is drawn toward the heat source.
- Purchase prechopped onions.

For the record, I always store my onions in the refrigerator, so they're always chilled when I chop them. I also chop rather quickly, so perhaps that helps, too. I always slice off the remaining root stem of the onion, then peel, then cut the onion in half lengthwise, then slice lengthwise. That's my method. May you find one that works for you.

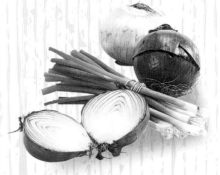

Jewel Yam Ramekins

▶ *Wheat-free. soy-free*

Though this dish can certainly be made in a large casserole pan, I like the idea of creating individual servings as a main or side dish.

2½ to 3 pounds (1138 to 1365 g) orange-fleshed garnet or jewel yams (about 4 large)

⅓ cup (80 ml) coconut milk

1 tablespoon (8 g) grated or minced fresh ginger

1 tablespoon (20 g) real maple syrup

½ teaspoon salt

⅓ cup (23 g) raw, unsweetened shredded coconut

2 tablespoons (30 ml) oil or melted nondairy butter (such as Earth Balance)

⅓ cup (42 g) toasted macadamia nuts, chopped

DIRECTIONS

Preheat the oven to 350°F (180°C, or gas mark 4). Lightly oil 4 or 6 ramekins or a single medium-sized casserole dish.

Poke a number of fork holes in each yam and bake for 1 to 1½ hours or until each is baked through. Times vary greatly depending on the size of your sweet potatoes; ultimately, you want the center of the yam to be as soft as the outer parts.

Remove the yams from the oven and let them cool for a few minutes so they're easy to handle. Remove the skin, which should easily peel off, and add the flesh to a blender or food processor.

Add the coconut milk and blend until creamy; then add the ginger, maple syrup, and salt and blend again. Taste and adjust the seasonings as needed.

Spoon the yam mixture into the prepared baking dishes, sprinkle with the coconut, drizzle with the oil, and bake uncovered until the coconut is golden and the mixture is warm throughout, 30 or 35 minutes. Remove from the oven, sprinkle with the toasted macadamia nuts, and serve hot.

YIELD: 4 to 6 servings

SERVING SUGGESTIONS AND VARIATIONS

Although the coconut milk imparts the richest flavor, other nondairy milks, such as almond and soy, work equally well.

PER SERVING: 421 Calories; 15g Fat (31.4% calories from fat); 5g Protein; 69g Carbohydrate; 11g Dietary Fiber; 0mg Cholesterol; 203mg Sodium

did you know?

What we call yams are actually not yams in the true sense. True yams are totally unrelated. However, for all intents and purposes, look for what are called "yams" in the grocery store: orange-fleshed tubers.

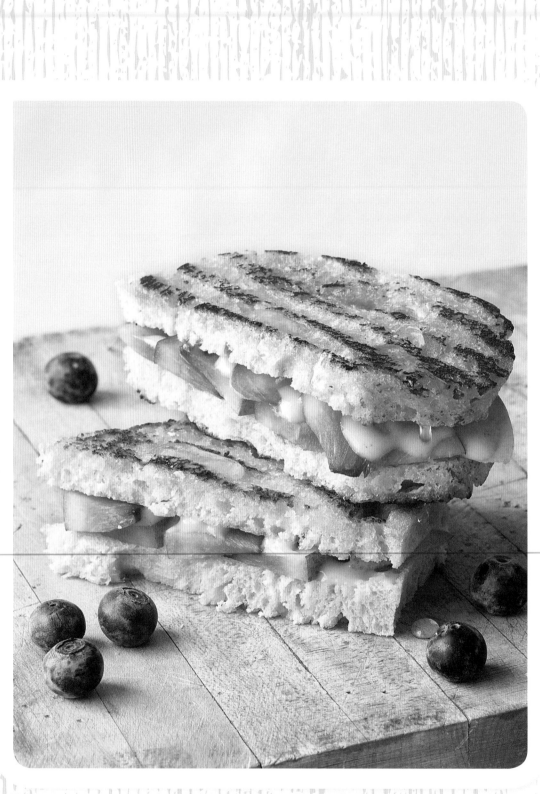

Nectarine Agave Panini

▶ *Soy-free if using soy-free Earth Balance and yogurt*

Panini—hot pressed sandwiches—are not just for savory meals! This is a healthful "dessert sandwich" that will inspire you to create other similar sweet concoctions.

1 container (6 ounces, or 170 g) nondairy yogurt (plain, vanilla, or fruit-based)

2 tablespoons (40 g) agave nectar, plus more for drizzling

¼ teaspoon pure vanilla extract

8 thin slices bread, crusts removed

2 ripe nectarines, peaches, or plums, unpeeled and thinly sliced

Ground cinnamon, for sprinkling

Light cooking spray or 3 tablespoons (42 g) nondairy butter (such as Earth Balance), divided

Blueberries or raspberries, for garnish

DIRECTIONS

Preheat your panini maker or use a sauté pan on the stove top.

In a small bowl, stir together the yogurt, agave, and vanilla until thoroughly combined. Carefully spread about 1 tablespoon (15 ml) of the yogurt mixture on one side of each of slices of bread. Arrange a layer of fruit over the yogurt, sprinkle on some cinnamon, and top with the remaining 4 slices of bread.

Lightly spray your preheated panini maker with a little cooking oil to ensure the sandwiches don't stick. Place 1 or 2 sandwiches (depending on the size of your machine) in the panini maker, press down, and cook for 4 minutes. Repeat with the remaining sandwiches.

If you aren't using a panini maker, melt 1 tablespoon (14 g) of the nondairy butter in a medium sauté pan over medium heat. Place 1 sandwich in the pan, place a flat heavy object on top, such as a cutting board, and cook for about 3 minutes on each side. Remove from the pan, transfer to a plate, and repeat with the remaining 2 tablespoons (28 g) butter and remaining 3 sandwiches.

Slice each sandwich in half on the diagonal, place on 4 dessert plates, drizzle with additional agave, and garnish with some blueberries. Serve immediately.

YIELD: 4 servings

SERVING SUGGESTIONS AND VARIATIONS

A versatile dish, these panini are appropriate as a unique dessert, akin to a sweet crepe, or as a sweet breakfast, not unlike a breakfast crepe.

PER SERVING: 284 Calories; 10g Fat (31.7% calories from fat); 5g Protein; 45g Carbohydrate; 3g Dietary Fiber; 0mg Cholesterol; 277mg Sodium

compassionate cooks' tips

- If you don't have a panini maker, you can also use a countertop electric grill.
- Quarter each sandwich on the diagonal for bite-size pieces.

advance preparation required

General Custard's Cream Pie with Almond Oat Crust

After serving this to friends Mark and Cheri Arellano on Christmas Day, I couldn't resist naming it what Mark blurted out upon tasting the first bite of this healthful version of cream pie.

1 cup (120 g) all-purpose flour

⅓ cup plus ¼ cup (65 g plus 50 g) granulated sugar, divided

¼ cup (35 g) coarsely ground almonds

¼ cup (20 g) rolled oats

Pinch of salt

½ cup (120 ml) canola oil or melted nondairy butter (such as Earth Balance)

1 cup (245 g) plain or vanilla nondairy yogurt

½ cup (115 g) extra-firm silken tofu

¼ cup (33 g) cornstarch mixed with 3 tablespoons (45 ml) water

¼ cup (60 ml) fresh orange juice

1 teaspoon pure vanilla extract

½ cup (150 g) apricot preserves, warmed

DIRECTIONS

Preheat the oven to 350°F (180°C, or gas mark 4). Lightly oil an 8-inch (20 cm) round pie pan.

In a large bowl, combine the flour, ⅓ cup (65 g) sugar, almonds, oats, and salt. Add the oil and stir until fully combined.

Transfer the flour mixture to the prepared pie pan and gently press the crust evenly over the bottom and up the sides of the pan to form a ½-inch-thick (2.5 cm) crust.

Bake the empty pie crust for 12 to 15 minutes or until lightly golden.

Meanwhile, in a blender or food processor, combine the yogurt, tofu, cornstarch mixture, remaining ¼ cup (50 g) sugar, orange juice, and vanilla and blend until smooth.

Remove the pie crust from the oven and pour the filling into the partially cooked crust. Bake for 35 to 40 minutes or until the filling is set but still slightly jiggly in the center. Let stand at room temperature for 10 minutes.

Pour the warm apricot preserves on top of the pie and gently spread in an even layer. Refrigerate until chilled, at least 2 hours. Using a warm knife, cut the pie into wedges and serve chilled or at room temperature.

YIELD: 8 to 10 servings

PER SERVING: 296 Calories; 14g Fat (41.9% calories from fat); 4g Protein; 40g Carbohydrate; 1g Dietary Fiber; 0mg Cholesterol; 38mg Sodium

compassionate cooks' tip

Add the leftover tofu to a fruit smoothie, blend it into a soup to add thickness, or use it to replace an egg in a baked good.

Persimmon Tea Cake

▶ *Soy-free if using soy-free Earth Balance*

This is a hearty, dense cake perfect for serving at a tea party or coffee klatch. It's even something that would stand up to a rum sauce and serve as a holiday dessert for grown-ups.

6 or 7 ripe Hachiya persimmons (see note)
½ cup (112 g) nondairy butter (such as Earth Balance), softened
1 cup (200 g) granulated sugar
1 tablespoon (15 ml) white or apple cider vinegar
1 teaspoon orange or lemon extract (optional)
2 cups (240 g) all-purpose flour
2 teaspoons baking powder
1 teaspoon baking soda
¼ teaspoon salt
½ teaspoon ground cinnamon
½ teaspoon ground nutmeg
½ teaspoon ground cloves
½ cup (65 g) chopped pecans or (60 g) walnuts
½ cup (75 g) raisins (optional)
1 teaspoon orange zest
½ teaspoon lemon zest
¼ cup (25 g) confectioners' sugar, for dusting

DIRECTIONS

Preheat the oven to 350°F (180°C, or gas mark 4). Lightly oil an 8 x 8-inch (20 x 20 cm) cake pan or Bundt pan.

Using a sharp knife, carefully peel the thin skin off the persimmons. Cut away any tough flesh or stems and transfer the flesh to a blender. (A food processor may not purée it as smoothly as needed.) Blend until puréed and then transfer to a large bowl.

Add the nondairy butter and sugar to the puréed persimmon pulp and cream together until fluffy. Add the vinegar and orange extract and stir until thoroughly combined.

In a separate bowl, stir together the flour, baking powder, baking soda, salt, cinnamon, nutmeg and cloves. Gradually blend the flour mixture into the persimmon mixture and stir in the nuts, raisins, orange zest, and lemon zest. The batter will be stiff, not thin. Spoon it into the prepared cake pan, and use a rubber spatula to even it out.

Bake for 35 to 40 minutes or until a toothpick inserted into the center comes out clean. Cool the cake in the pan for 10 minutes and turn out onto a rack to continue cooling an additional 20 minutes before serving. Sprinkle with confectioners' sugar, and serve.

YIELD: 12 servings

PER SERVING: 284 Calories; 11g Fat (33.9% calories from fat); 3g Protein; 45g Carbohydrate; 2g Dietary Fiber; 0mg Cholesterol; 232mg Sodium

compassionate cooks' tips

- Hachiya, the taller persimmon, is the best type to use for this recipe, because as it ripens, it becomes very soft and jellylike. The Fuyu is the squat, short persimmon that retains its crispiness and would not work here.

- Once you purée the pulp, you can transfer it to an airtight container and freeze for up to 3 months.

- The jellylike pulp of the Hachiya persimmon is also great for adding to fruit smoothies, as a topping for nondairy ice cream, and as an addition to fruit salsa.

Mango Papaya Punch

▶ *Soy-free, wheat-free, oil-free*

A refreshing hot-weather beverage, this punch provides oodles more nutrition than any store-bought juice.

1 cup (175 g) frozen mango chunks
1 cup (140 g) frozen papaya chunks
1 cup (235 ml) fresh orange juice
¼ cup (60 ml) lime juice (from 1 medium lime)
3 to 4 cups (705 to 940 ml) cold water, or to desired thickness
1 teaspoon grated orange zest
Crushed ice, for serving
Fresh mint leaves, for garnish

DIRECTIONS

Place the mango and papaya in a blender. Cover and purée until smooth. Add the orange juice, lime juice, water, and orange zest. Blend well and taste. Serve over crushed ice in pretty glasses and garnish with fresh mint leaves.

YIELD: 8 servings

SERVING SUGGESTIONS AND VARIATIONS

Serve in a chilled, sugar-rimmed glass

PER SERVING: 35 Calories; trace Fat (2.0% calories from fat); trace Protein; 9g Carbohydrate; 1g Dietary Fiber; 0mg Cholesterol; 4mg Sodium

compassionate cooks' tips

- Some testers for this recipe opted for a slightly sweeter version and so added a few tablespoons (26 to 39 g) of sugar when blending the fruit. Agave nectar would also work well.

- Although you can certainly use fresh fruit, frozen tends to add the thickness and cold that makes this a special punch. If you choose to cut up your own fruit, perhaps throw them in the freezer for an hour before proceeding with the recipe

WAYS TO INCREASE ORANGE FOODS

- Add orange zest to main dishes, side dishes, or salads.

- Add orange, nectarine, or mandarin wedges to salad.

- When making or buying fresh orange juice, choose the kind with the pulp.

- Add edible orange flowers, such as nasturtiums, marigolds, and chrysanthemums, to green salads.

- Start the day with a glass of orange juice for breakfast.

- Instead of potato french fries, bake sweet potato slices or carrot fries (see page 59 for recipe).

- Snack on dried apricot, mango, and papaya.

- Add yams or sweet potatoes to bean chili or bean burritos.

- Make an orange fruit salad of papaya, orange wedges, cantaloupe, apricots, and peaches.

- Snack on carrot sticks.

- Bake a sweet potato instead of a yellow potato.

- Add sliced orange bell peppers to a stir-fry or salad.

- Grill chunks of orange bell peppers on a kabob or roast whole.

- Try orange tomatoes for a change.

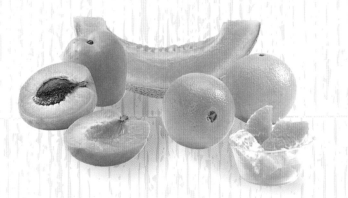

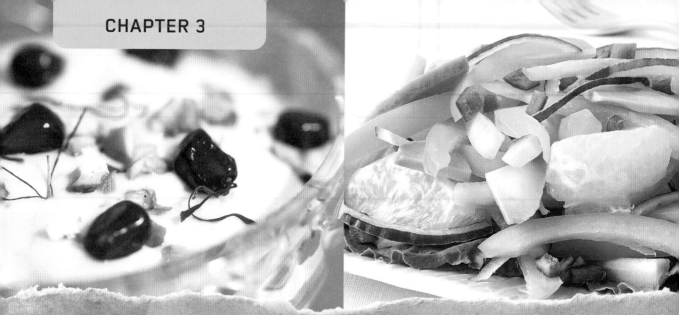

color me
YeLLow

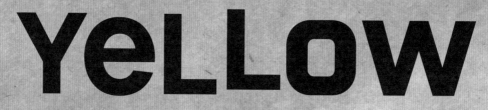

LET THE SUNSHINE IN

Yellow flowers may very well be my favorite. They just shout a joyous "spring is here!" and make it impossible to be unhappy in their presence. I'm thinking of yellow tulips, daisies, dahlias, black-eyed Susans, sunflowers, orchids, narcissus, and even the common dandelion.

When it comes to yellow fruits and vegetables, most of them are indeed associated with spring as well as summer, such as corn, pineapples, lemons, mangoes, summer squash, yellow bell peppers, bananas, and grapefruit.

What all these plants—the flowers as well as the fruits—share is a carotenoid called zeaxanthin, which gives many of them their characteristic yellow hue. In addition, zeaxanthin breaks down to form *picrocrocin* and *safranal* (responsible for the taste and aroma of saffron).

Lutein

Another carotenoid that makes itself known in yellow (as well as orange and green plant foods) is lutein (pronounced LOO-teen). Its name, in fact, comes from the Latin word *luteus*, which means "yellow." Although we tend to associate beta-carotene with eye health, lutein is one of the main antioxidants in the eye and works with zeaxanthin to prevent such diseases as age-related macular degeneration, the leading cause of blindness in people over fifty.

I find it perplexing that some people recommend chicken's eggs for their concentrations of lutein in the yellow yolk. Although with eggs you also consume saturated fat, dietary cholesterol, and unhealthful and unnecessary animal protein, the only reason you consume lutein through eggs is because the chickens ate lutein, an antioxidant derived from plants.

Commercially, lutein is used in chicken feed to provide the yellow color of broiler chicken skin as well as a darker yellow egg yolk. Polled consumers viewed yellow chicken skin more favorably than white chicken skin. Today, using lutein to deepen the color of egg yolks is the main reason chicken feed is fortified. This just emphasizes my point that the nutrients we need are *plant-based*. To go *through* animals to get the nutrients *they* got from plants makes absolutely no sense, though it does make a lot of money. The lutein market is a multimillion dollar industry, whether it's used in pharmaceuticals, animal feed, or human food.

And though it's true that the lutein in egg yolks is more *bioavailable* (our bodies absorb and use it effectively), it's not the egg yolks themselves that make this possible but rather the *fat* in the yolk. In other words, plant-based fats would just as effectively (and more healthfully) increase the bioavailability of lutein. So, just as I recommended in the introduction to the orange chapter (page 45), I recommend eating lutein-rich foods with a little fat. Lutein-rich foods that include a little fat in this section are Corn Chowder (page 83), Spicy Yellow Bell Pepper Soup (page 85), and Creamed Corn (page 88). If you tend not to cook with oil, then add some healthful nuts or seeds as a garnish.

Pineapple Mango Chutney

▶ *Oil-free if using water to sauté, soy-free, wheat-free*

Use this incredibly flavorful and beautiful dish as a "salsa" for the Indian-Style Black Bean and Veggie Burritos (page 238), a topping for rice, or the basis for a vegetable stir-fry. Sweet tropical fruit always pairs well with spicy flavors, such as hot peppers and ginger, as I've done here.

2 tablespoons (30 ml) oil or water, for sautéing
1 teaspoon crushed red pepper flakes
1 large yellow onion, minced
1 tablespoon (6 g) minced fresh ginger
1 large yellow bell pepper, diced
2 ripe mangoes, peeled and diced
1 small pineapple, peeled and diced
¼ cup (60 g) firmly packed brown sugar
1½ tablespoons (9.5 g) curry powder
½ cup (120 ml) apple cider vinegar

DIRECTIONS

Heat the oil in a large sauté pan over medium heat. Stir in the red pepper flakes, cook until they begin to sizzle, about 1 minute, and then add the minced onion. Reduce the heat to low and cook, stirring occasionally, until the onion has softened, about 7 minutes. (This process is faster with oil, slower with water.)

Increase the heat to medium and stir in the ginger, bell pepper, mangoes, pineapple, brown sugar, curry powder, and vinegar. Bring to a simmer and cook for 25 to 30 minutes, stirring occasionally. Cool the chutney completely when done and store in airtight containers in the refrigerator.

YIELD: 32 servings, about 2 tablespoons (30 g) each

SERVING SUGGESTIONS AND VARIATIONS

• Divide the chutney among several clear jars, add a ribbon, and give as a gift.
• Serve chutney over brown rice, on lentils, or in wraps—whatever your imagination concocts.

PER SERVING: 31 Calories; 1g Fat (24.5% calories from fat); trace Protein; 6g Carbohydrate; 1g Dietary Fiber; 0mg Cholesterol; 1mg Sodium

food lore

Next to bananas, pineapple is the second most popular tropical fruit. Pineapples contain a mixture of enzymes called bromelain, which reduces inflammation, making it helpful for treating arthritis, gout, sore throat, and acute sinusitis.

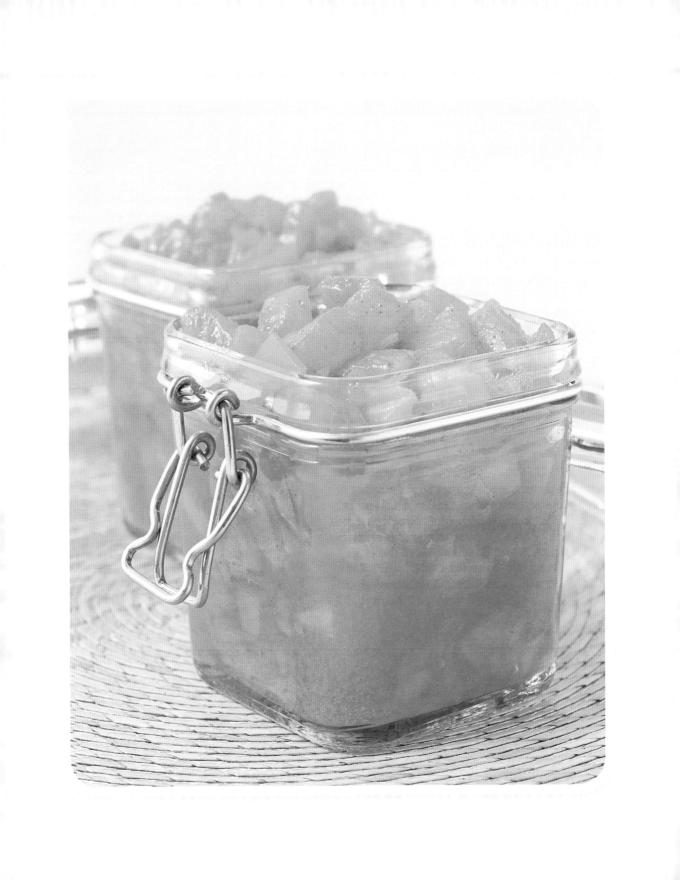

advance preparation required

Lemon Basil Vinaigrette

▶ *Wheat-free, soy-free*

Light and creamy at the same time, this dressing is perfect for any combination of mixed greens.

¼ cup (60 ml) olive oil

2 tablespoons (30 ml) fresh lemon juice

2 tablespoons (30 ml) fresh orange juice

Zest from 1 lemon

¼ teaspoon salt

1 tablespoon (20 g) agave nectar

¼ cup (10 g) finely chopped fresh basil

1 teaspoon white wine or apple cider vinegar

Salt and freshly ground pepper, to taste

DIRECTIONS

In a jar with a lid or in the pitcher of your blender, combine the olive oil, lemon juice, orange juice, lemon zest, salt, agave, basil, and vinegar. Seal and shake well or turn on the blender. Taste and adjust the seasonings with salt and pepper, as necessary.

Chill for at least 2 hours in the refrigerator. Strain the basil before serving, if desired.

YIELD: 5 servings, about 2 tablespoons (30 ml) each

SERVING SUGGESTIONS AND VARIATIONS

- Modify this recipe by using any combination of citrus you have on hand, including grapefruit, tangerines, or limes.
- Toss with mixed baby greens, dried cranberries, tangerine wedges, and toasted pecans; mix with romaine lettuce, pear tomatoes, and halved grapes; or pour over arugula, spinach, walnuts, and red onion slices.

compassionate cooks' tip

Some testers liked to strain the basil before serving the dressing; some preferred the basil to remain in the dressing.

PER SERVING: 119 Calories; 11g Fat (80.3% calories from fat); trace Protein; 6g Carbohydrate; 1g Dietary Fiber; 0mg Cholesterol; 107mg Sodium

TASTE THE ONION RAINBOW

Perhaps the most common vegetable used in a variety of cuisines, onion adds an abundance of flavor, color, and nutrition to any dish. Containing more than 150 phytochemicals, onions have varying flavors depending on the type. Keep in mind that the stronger the flavor, the more protective organo-sulfur compounds they contain. Another anticancer phytochemical abundant in the stronger-flavored onions is quercetin, found in yellow and red onions, as well as shallots. White onions, though they are more mild-tasting for sensitive palates, lack this antioxidant. Below is a guide to help you choose from the many varieties.

Yellow: This is a versatile onion appropriate for a variety of uses, but most people find it too pungent to be eaten raw (except me!). Because it's higher in the sulfur-based compounds, it has a more complex flavor, as well as more nutrition, than do white onions. Yellow onions become sweeter and milder when cooked, thus making them perfect for caramelizing.
Alternatives: Sweet or white onions

Sweet: Although they are fine for cooking, their mild and sweet flavor makes them perfect as a burger topping or sandwich filling. The most popular sweet onion is the Vidalia, but there are other varieties, such as Walla Walla, Sweet Imperial, Texas Spring Sweet, Arizona, and Maui.
Alternatives: Red onion or bulbs of green onions

White: A popular cooking onion, it is often used in herbed, spicy dishes, such as those in Mexican cuisine, because of its clean flavor. White onions tend to be sweeter than yellow onions, but because of their higher water content, they are more prone to mold and should be stored in the refrigerator.
Alternatives: Yellow or sweet onions

Green: Green onions (known as scallions) are called shallots in Australia and spring onions in Britain. These are onions with small bulbs and long green stalks. They are usually eaten raw, but also can be grilled or sautéed.
Alternatives: Spring onions, leeks, shallots, or chives

Red/Purple: Sweet enough to be eaten raw, red onions are often added to salads and are delicious grilled. Because the anthocyanin pigments are related to quercetin, red/purple onions have higher amounts, thus increasing their antioxidant protection.
Alternatives: Green onions (in salads); sweet or white onions (when cooking)

Cashew Cheese

▶ *Wheat-free*

I included this fabulous cheese in *The Vegan Table*, based on the recipe in *The Real Food Daily Cookbook* by Ann Gentry. I'm including it here again as a slicing cheese but also for the Swiss Chard Pie (page 93). For the former, the cheese should include agar (see variations below) to set it up so it can be sliced for crackers; for the latter, it should be kept creamy.

1¼ cups (188 g) raw cashews

½ cup (72 g) nutritional yeast

2 teaspoons onion powder

1 to 2 teaspoons salt, to taste

1 teaspoon garlic powder

⅛ teaspoon ground white pepper

3½ cups (823 ml) nondairy milk (such as almond, soy, rice, hazelnut, hemp, or oat)

3 tablespoons (24 g) cornstarch (or agar flakes—see note below)

½ cup (120 ml) canola oil

¼ cup (63 g) light (yellow or white) miso paste

2 tablespoons (30 ml) fresh lemon juice (about 1 lemon)

DIRECTIONS

Add the cashews to the large bowl of a food processor and using the pulse button, finely grind the cashews. Don't allow the cashews to turn into a paste. Add the nutritional yeast, onion powder, salt, garlic powder, and white pepper. Pulse three more times to blend in the spices.

Combine the milk, cornstarch, and oil in a heavy saucepan. Bring to a simmer over high heat. Decrease the heat to low-medium, cover, and simmer, stirring occasionally, for 10 minutes or until the cornstarch is dissolved.

With the food processor running, gradually add the milk/oil mixture to the cashew/nutritional yeast mixture. Blend for 2 minutes or until very smooth and creamy. Next, blend in the miso and lemon juice.

The cheese will keep for 4 days, covered and refrigerated.

YIELD: 32 servings, about 2 tablespoons (30 g) each

SERVING SUGGESTIONS AND VARIATIONS

The cheese you prepare using this recipe will be creamy, perfect for macaroni and cheese or as a sauce for vegetables. If you would like to make a hard block of cheese, substitute the cornstarch for 1 cup (about 2 ounces, or 55 g) of agar flakes. Transfer the creamy mixture to the type of container that you want it molded to (rectangular, square, or round). Once it sets up (after a few hours in the refrigerator), unmold it, and slice or grate it.

PER SERVING: 75 Calories; 6g Fat (66.0% calories from fat); 3g Protein; 4g Carbohydrate; 1g Dietary Fiber; 0mg Cholesterol; 230mg Sodium

THE POWER OF POTATOES

Most people don't think of potatoes when they think of adding color to their diets, but perhaps they should. The potato tends to get a bad rap, mostly because people think only of the starchy white potato when they think of these popular tubers, but there are a variety of other colors whose nutrition profile changes according to the potato type and color: red, yellow, orange, purple, and blue. (See Potato Varieties, page 148.)

In 2005, Europeans consumed almost 65 million tons of potatoes, North Americans consumed almost 20 million tons (17 million in the U.S. alone), and world consumption in the same year topped out at almost 203 million tons.

Unfortunately, most of these potatoes are consumed in the form of french fries or potato chips, and when they're eaten whole, they're mostly the starchy white variety, often drowned in dairy-based butter. But this doesn't have to be the case. Potatoes can be a healthful part of our diets, especially when we explore other colors and methods of preparation. Consider this:

- Yellow potatoes contain carotenoids in both their flesh and their skin. The antioxidants vary according to the intensity of the color and are primarily lutein, zeaxanthin, and violaxanthin. (See page 22 for more information.)

- Deeply yellow or orange flesh potatoes, such as sweet potatoes, have levels of carotenoids similar to those in winter squash.

- The antioxidants in red-skinned potatoes are found primarily in the skins. However, in the less familiar purple varieties, the antioxidants—in this case, anthocyanins—are in both the skin and the flesh, increasing their nutrient density.

- The purple-blue pigment anthocyanin is saturated in the potato whose flesh and skin are both purple. Some purple potatoes have purple skin but a lighter color flesh.

- The most healthful preparations for potatoes are those that lock the nutrients in and keep the whole vegetable intact. For instance, though peeling once in a while is fine when you want the texture to be smooth and creamy, try to consume the peel as often as possible.

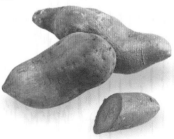

- Roasting and steaming are my favorite ways of cooking potatoes: a little olive oil, a little salt, and you're good to go.

Grapefruit, Yellow Pepper, and Avocado Salad

▶ *Wheat-free, soy-free*

"An explosion of yin and yang," said one of the enthusiastic testers of this recipe: creamy from the avocado, sour from the grapefruit, sweet from the agave, cool and crunchy from the cucumber and lettuce, and hot from the red onion and jalapeño.

1 large yellow grapefruit, peeled and
    separated into wedges

2 yellow bell peppers, sliced

2 medium cucumbers, peeled, seeded, and
    cut into 1-inch (2.5 cm) matchsticks

1 medium red onion, sliced

1 tablespoon (15 ml) olive oil

1 tablespoon (20 g) agave nectar

1 jalapeño pepper, minced

¼ teaspoon salt

2 ripe avocados, halved, pitted, and sliced

8 romaine lettuce leaves, left whole

Freshly ground pepper, to taste

DIRECTIONS

In a bowl, combine the grapefruit wedges, peppers, cucumber, and onion.

In a small bowl, combine the oil, agave, minced jalapeño, and salt. Pour over the grapefruit mixture and toss to combine.

Add the avocado slices and gently toss, avoiding mashing the avocado. Serve right away or marinate for 1 hour.

When ready to serve, divide the whole romaine lettuce leaves among 4 plates. Top each with the marinated mixture and grind some fresh pepper over the top.

YIELD: 4 servings

SERVING SUGGESTIONS AND VARIATIONS

• Use jicama in place of or in addition to the cucumber.

• Pink grapefruit can most certainly be substituted for the yellow grapefruit.

• If you dont like peppers, use yellow (or red) tomatoes instead

PER SERVING: 269 Calories; 19g Fat (59.2% calories from fat); 4g Protein; 26g Carbohydrate; 6g Dietary Fiber; 0mg Cholesterol; 151mg Sodium

compassionate cooks' tip

If you don't like it too spicy, seed the jalapeño pepper first.

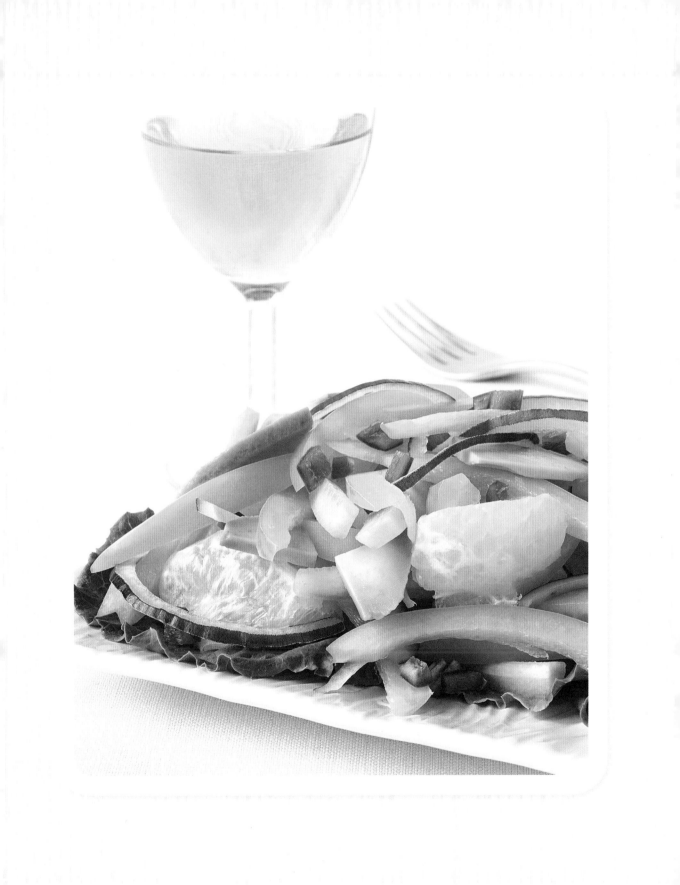

Curried Cauliflower Soup

▶ *Oil-free, wheat-free, soy-free*

This soup's secret ingredient—an apple—lends a touch of tangy sweetness that complements the curry's spice. Letting the soup cool for 20 minutes before blending helps deepen the flavors.

2 tablespoons (30 ml) water, for sautéing
1 yellow onion, chopped
1 medium tart apple, peeled, cored, and
    coarsely chopped
1 tablespoon (6 g) curry powder
1 clove garlic, minced
1 large head cauliflower, chopped into
    uniform-size pieces
4 cups (940 ml) vegetable stock
Salt, to taste

DIRECTIONS
Heat the water in a soup pot over medium-high heat. Add the onion and sauté for 5 to 7 minutes or until soft and translucent. Stir in the apple, curry powder, and garlic and cook for 2 minutes longer or until the curry powder turns a deep yellow. Add a little more water as necessary to keep the contents from sticking to the bottom of the pot.

Add the cauliflower and vegetable stock and bring to a simmer. Cover, reduce the heat to medium-low, and simmer for 20 minutes. Cool for 20 minutes and then blend in a food processor or blender until smooth. Season with salt and serve.

YIELD: 6 servings

SERVING SUGGESTIONS AND VARIATIONS
Using a blender to purée the soup will yield a smoother, creamier soup than one puréed using a food processor.

PER SERVING: 39 Calories; 1g Fat (18.9% calories from fat); 1g Protein; 8g Carbohydrate; 2g Dietary Fiber; 0mg Cholesterol; 669mg Sodium

did you know?

Used in many Indian dishes, *curry* is actually a generic term that refers to the combination of spices it typically comprises: cumin, coriander, fenugreek, and especially turmeric, which gives curry its characteristic deep yellow hue. With an earthy, bitter, peppery flavor and a mustardy smell, turmeric is known for its main phytochemical, *curcumin*, which has anticancer, antioxidant, and anti-inflammatory properties. In fact, turmeric has been used for thousands of years in traditional Ayurvedic medicine in India as a treatment for arthritis, autoimmune diseases, and heart disease.

food lore

In medieval Europe, turmeric was known as Indian saffron, because it is widely used as an alternative to the far more expensive saffron spice. For that reason, it's also called "poor man's saffron."

Corn Chowder

▶ *Wheat-free, soy-free if using soy-free milk and oil for sautéing*

A perfect dish when corn is abundant in the summer months, this chowder also provides cozy comfort in the colder seasons, when frozen corn can be used instead.

2 teaspoons nondairy butter (such as Earth Balance) or oil

3 cups (465 g) corn kernels, fresh or frozen

1 tablespoon (15 ml) oil or water, for sautéing

1 yellow onion, roughly chopped

1 yellow potato, such as Yukon Gold, peeled and cubed

4 cups (940 ml) vegetable stock

1 cup (235 ml) nondairy milk (such as almond, soy, rice, hazelnut, hemp, or oat)

Salt and freshly ground pepper, to taste

1 large tomato, seeded and finely chopped, for garnish

3 tablespoons (7.5 g) chopped fresh basil leaves, for garnish

DIRECTIONS

Heat the butter in a large sauté pan over medium heat. Add the corn and cook for 15 to 20 minutes until the corn begins to brown a bit. Alternatively, you may grill or roast the corn.

Meanwhile, heat the oil in a large soup pot over medium heat. Add the onion and sauté until the onion is translucent, about 5 minutes. Add the potato and stock and bring to a boil. Reduce the heat to low, cover, and cook until the potato cubes are tender, about 20 minutes.

Once the potatoes can be pierced with a fork and the corn is finished browning, add the corn to the pot with the potatoes and cook for 10 minutes.

Ladle 2 cups (470 ml) of the soup into a food processor or blender and process until smooth. (You may also use an immersion blender, puréeing only some of the soup and leaving the rest chunky.)

Add the puréed portion back into the pot and add the milk. Heat just to warm it up, season with salt and pepper to taste, and ladle the soup into bowls. Garnish with the tomato and basil and serve.

YIELD: 4 servings

PER SERVING: 235 Calories; 9g Fat (30.1% calories from fat); 7g Protein; 38g Carbohydrate; 5g Dietary Fiber; 0mg Cholesterol; 1014mg Sodium

did you know?

Corn is rich in folate, a B vitamin that prevents birth defects. Folate is the naturally occurring substance in plants; folic acid is the synthetic form used for supplements. Folate helps lower levels of homocysteine, an amino acid that can damage blood vessels, increasing the risk of heart attacks and strokes. One cup (155 g) of corn supplies almost 20 percent of the Daily Value for folate.

compassionate cooks' tip

Three cups (465 g) of corn equals 4 medium ears.

Yellow Split Pea Soup with Collard Greens and Yams

▶ *Oil-free, soy-free, wheat-free*

This slight variation on traditional split pea soup packs a super antioxidant punch with the yellow turmeric, green collards, and orange yams.

2 tablespoons (30 ml) water, for sautéing
2 yellow onions, coarsely chopped
1 tablespoon (6 g) minced fresh ginger
3 cloves garlic, minced
1½ to 2 tablespoons (9 to 12 g) curry powder
1 teaspoon ground cumin
½ teaspoon ground mustard
½ teaspoon turmeric
1 medium or 2 small garnet or jewel yams, peeled and cut into 1-inch (2.5 cm) cubes
1 medium carrot, diced (peeling optional)
8 cups (1880 ml) vegetable stock (homemade or store-bought)
3 cups (420 g) dried yellow split peas, picked over and rinsed
1 bunch collard greens, chopped into bite-size pieces
1 teaspoon salt, or to taste
Freshly ground pepper, to taste

DIRECTIONS

Heat the water in a large soup pot and add the onions. Stir and cook until they turn translucent, about 7 minutes. Add the ginger and garlic and cook for 5 more minutes, adding any additional water to prevent them from sticking to the bottom of the pot.

Add the curry powder, cumin, mustard, turmeric, yams, carrot, stock, and split peas to the pot. Stir to combine.

Cover and simmer until the split peas are tender and broken down, about 1 hour. Stir often to make sure the split peas don't stick to the bottom of the pot.

About 10 minutes before the soup is done, add the chopped collard greens to the pot, stir to combine, and cook for about 10 minutes until they soften and integrate with the rest of the soup. Season with salt, to taste, and serve hot with freshly ground pepper.

YIELD: 6 to 8 servings

SERVING SUGGESTIONS AND VARIATIONS

- Use any leafy green, such as kale or chard, in place of the collards.
- To freeze, let the soup cool completely before adding to a freezer-safe container.
- Purée 2 cups (470 ml) of the cooked soup before adding the greens and return it to the soup to add even more thickness. Add the greens and continue with the recipe.

PER SERVING: 246 Calories; 2g Fat (7.2% calories from fat); 14g Protein; 45g Carbohydrate; 16g Dietary Fiber; 0mg Cholesterol; 1276mg Sodium

Spicy Yellow Bell Pepper Soup

▶ *Wheat-free, soy-free, oil-free if sautéing in water*

You can make this soup even more colorful by making a second batch with roasted red bell peppers and pouring the yellow and red soups into the serving bowls at the same time.

1 tablespoon (15 ml) oil or water, for sautéing

1 large yellow onion, coarsely chopped

4 large yellow bell peppers, cut into 1-inch (2.5 cm) pieces

1 or 2 jalapeño peppers, seeded and chopped

1 large yellow potato (½ pound, or 225 g), peeled and cut into ½-inch (1.3 cm) pieces

4 cups (940 ml) vegetable stock

Salt, to taste

2 tablespoons (30 ml) sherry or red wine vinegar

2 tablespoons (8 g) chopped cilantro or (8 g) parsley

DIRECTIONS

In a soup pot, heat the oil. Add the onion, yellow bell peppers, and jalapeños and cook over medium-low heat, stirring occasionally, until the vegetables begin to soften, about 7 minutes.

Add the potato, vegetable stock, and salt to taste. Bring to a boil, cover partially, and reduce the heat to a simmer. Cook until the vegetables are tender, about 25 minutes.

Purée the soup in a blender or food processor or use an immersion blender until smooth. You may need to work in batches if your blender or food processor is on the small side.

Return the soup to the pot and reheat gently. Stir in the vinegar and season with salt. Ladle the soup into shallow bowls, top with the chopped cilantro, and serve.

YIELD: 6 servings

PER SERVING: 90 Calories; 3g Fat (31.9% calories from fat); 2g Protein; 14g Carbohydrate; 2g Dietary Fiber; 0mg Cholesterol; 666mg Sodium

food lore

Native to Central and South America, the "bell pepper" goes by many names depending on where you are in the world:

- In Great Britain, it is called a "pepper," whereas in countries such as Australia, India, Malaysia, and New Zealand, they are called "capsicum."

- Across Europe, it may be called "paprika," whose etymological roots are in the word *pepper*. (Of course, "paprika" refers to the powdered spice made from the same fruit.)

- In the United States and Canada, it is referred to simply as a "pepper" or referred to by color (e.g., "red pepper," "green pepper").

- In Denmark, the bell pepper is referred to as *peberfrugt*, meaning "pepper-fruit."

compassionate cooks' tip

The soup can be refrigerated for up to 2 days.

ARE ANTIOXIDANT SUPPLEMENTS SAFE?

According to the *Journal of the American Medical Association (JAMA)*, 10 to 20 percent of the adult population of North America and Europe (80 to 160 million people) consume antioxidant supplements. Recently, a group of researchers thoroughly examined the effects of antioxidant supplements in terms of mortality. The results were published in a recent issue of JAMA, in which the authors reported, "We did not find convincing evidence that antioxidant supplements have beneficial effects on mortality. Even more, beta-carotene, vitamin A, and vitamin E seem to increase the risk of death. Further randomized trials are needed to establish the effects of vitamin C and selenium."

In this detailed analysis, a total of 232,606 people in 68 trials were examined. Looking at beta-carotene, vitamin A, and vitamin E singly or in combinations, they found that people who take these antioxidant supplements don't live any longer than those who don't take them. The research also shows no benefit—but also no harm—for vitamin C supplements. Selenium supplements tended to very slightly reduce risk of death.

The most significant take-away from this report is that the researchers emphasized that their findings should not be translated to potential effects of *fruits and vegetables*. They wanted to make it clear that they were talking about synthetic supplements, not the naturally occurring antioxidants in plants.

Vitamin A

Based on the analysis, the researches found that people who take vitamin A supplements have an *increased* risk of death. The recommendation for vitamin A is 5,000 IUs, and most multivitamins probably contain that many. More important, an abundance of plant foods contains hundreds of carotenoids (one of which is beta-carotene, which our bodies convert into vitamin A). So pile on the sweet potatoes, carrots, kale, mango, spinach, turnip greens, winter squash, collard greens, cilantro, and fresh thyme and consume your vitamin A and carotenoids naturally.

Vitamin E

The findings show that there is no evidence that vitamin E supplements are beneficial, and in fact, there is a hint that they may be harmful. The RDA for vitamin E is just 15 milligrams (about 23 IU) a day. The upper limit is 1,000 milligrams (about 1,500 IU) a day. For a while, professionals were recommending taking vitamin E supplements because of its efficacy in reducing heart disease and cancer, but whereas vitamin E from foods does this, nearly all the clinical trials on vitamin E supplements from the past few years have yielded negative, inconclusive, or neutral results. Bottom line: get vitamin E from food.

The best food sources of vitamin E are mustard greens, turnip greens, collard greens, kale, chard, spinach, almonds, and sunflower seeds. Also great are olives, avocado, wheat germ, Brussels sprouts, asparagus, and other nuts and seeds. Keep in mind that the RDA for vitamin E is 15 milligrams for adults, and 1 ounce (28 g) of raw almonds has almost 7 milligrams, one medium avocado has about 2.5, and one medium sweet potato has almost 6, so just from those foods alone, you will not have a problem getting your vitamin E from foods.

Vitamin C

Although the researchers concluded that there isn't anything harmful about taking vitamin C supplements, they also found there is no real benefit, and you might be able to put your money to better use by getting your vitamin C from food. The RDA is a mere 90 milligrams for adult males and 75 for adult females.

The best sources of vitamin C are broccoli, bell peppers, kale, cauliflower, strawberries, lemons, mustard and turnip greens, Brussels sprouts, papaya, chard, cabbage, spinach, kiwifruit, snow peas, cantaloupe, oranges, grapefruit, limes, tomatoes, zucchini, raspberries, asparagus, celery, pineapples, lettuce, watermelon, fennel, peppermint, and parsley. Just ½ cup (75 g) of chopped raw bell pepper contains about 140 milligrams of vitamin C, 1 cup (110 g) of whole strawberries contains 82 milligrams, one medium orange has 70 milligrams, and ½ cup (40 g) of cooked broccoli has 58 milligrams.

Zinc and Selenium

Although there appears to be no harm in taking selenium and zinc supplements, there appears to be no benefit either. The RDA for zinc is 11 milligrams a day for men and 8 milligrams for women. For children 7 months to 3 years, it's 3 milligrams; for children 4 to 8, it's 5 milligrams; and for children 9 to 13, it's 8 milligrams. The RDA for pregnant and lactating women is 13 and 14 milligrams, respectively.

Cashews, chickpeas, vegetarian baked beans, and pecans all come in at about 1.5 milligrams for small amounts, so again, you'll have no problem finding zinc in your food.

Creamed Corn

▶ *Wheat-free*

Admittedly, I grew up eating cream corn from a can, and even though many brands are technically "vegan," they're full of artificial ingredients. Opt, instead, for this quick homemade version.

2 packages (10 ounces, or 280 g) frozen corn kernels, thawed (or the equivalent fresh)

2 tablespoons (28 g) nondairy butter (such as Earth Balance)

1 tablespoon (13 g) granulated sugar

1 teaspoon salt

¼ teaspoon freshly ground black pepper

1½ cups (353 ml) nondairy milk (such as almond, soy, rice, hazelnut, hemp, or oat)

4 teaspoons (11 g) cornstarch

DIRECTIONS

In a sauté pan over medium-high heat, sauté the corn in the butter for about 5 minutes. Reduce the heat and add the sugar, salt, and pepper.

In a separate bowl or measuring cup, whisk together the milk and cornstarch and stir into the corn mixture. Cook, stirring, over low-medium heat, until the mixture is thickened and the corn is heated through, 10 to 15 minutes.

Remove from the heat and serve hot.

YIELD: 4 servings

PER SERVING: 162 Calories; 7g Fat (38.7% calories from fat); 5g Protein; 22g Carbohydrate; 3g Dietary Fiber; 0mg Cholesterol; 546mg Sodium

did you know?

Lutein and zeaxanthin, both members of the carotenoid family, are the pigments that give corn its yellow hue. In addition to fighting heart disease and cancer, these antioxidants also appear to protect a sensitive area of the eye called the macula, which enables to us to make out the fine features of an object. Though macular degeneration is the leading cause of blindness in older adults, research findings suggest that it may be prevented with the help of lutein and zeaxanthin.

Ginger-Roasted Parsnips

▶ *Wheat-free, soy-free*

Parsnips tend to be underrated, but I confess, I love the earthiness of these root vegetables. To keep the ginger from burning, I suggest a slow "roast" in a lower-than-normal oven.

2 tablespoons (30 ml) olive oil
1¼ pounds (570 g) parsnips, peeled and
   coarsely chopped
1½ tablespoons (9 g) minced fresh ginger
Salt and freshly ground pepper, to taste

PER SERVING: 159 Calories; 7g Fat (39.8% calories from fat); 2g Protein; 23g Carbohydrate; 6g Dietary Fiber; 0mg Cholesterol; 13mg Sodium

DIRECTIONS

Preheat the oven to 325°F (170°C, or gas mark 3).

Pour the olive oil into a 9 x 13-inch (23 x 33 cm) baking dish, preferably glass.

Add the parsnips and ginger, season with salt and pepper, and toss to coat with the oil and seasonings. Cover, and bake for 40 minutes until the parsnips are tender.

Adjust the seasonings, as necessary, and serve right away.

YIELD: 4 servings

SERVING SUGGESTIONS AND VARIATIONS

Add carrots along with the parsnips (and perhaps a little extra oil and ginger).

compassionate cooks' tips

- The parsnips can be roasted up to 4 hours ahead. Reheat, covered, in a 350°F (180°C, or gas mark 4) oven.

- It doesn't matter what size or shape you cut the parsnips before they cook as long as they are all uniform size so they cook evenly.

- Seven medium parsnips weigh approximately 1¼ pounds (570 g).

- Parsnips look like fatter, beige versions of carrots and can be treated just as the more popular orange root vegetables are: baked, boiled, roasted, puréed, or fried.

Summer Squash with Cherry Tomatoes Topped with Cheesy Toasted Pine Nuts

▶ *Wheat-free, soy-free*

This is a favorite in our household when our zucchini squash and Sun Gold tomatoes are overflowing in our garden.

1½ pounds (683 g) green and/or yellow summer
  squash, cut into ½-inch (1.3 cm) cubes
2 to 3 tablespoons (30 to 45 ml) olive oil
1 tablespoon (4 g) minced fresh parsley
1 tablespoon (4 g) minced fresh basil
1 tablespoon (4 g) minced fresh thyme
4 or 5 cloves garlic, peeled and minced
  (or more!)
2 cups (300 g) cherry tomatoes, stemmed
  and halved
Salt and freshly ground pepper, to taste
¼ cup (35 g) toasted pine nuts
1 tablespoon (6 g) nutritional yeast

DIRECTIONS

Preheat the oven to 375°F (190°C, or gas mark 5).

Combine the squash, oil, herbs, and garlic in a large bowl and toss to combine. Add the tomatoes and salt and pepper to taste and toss gently. Set aside.

Add the pine nuts, nutritional yeast, and salt to taste to the food processor and process until the pine nuts are crumbled and thoroughly combined with the nutritional yeast and salt.

Transfer the vegetable mixture to a 9 x 9-inch or 9 x 13-inch (23 x 23 cm or 23 x 33 cm) glass casserole pan, and spoon the pine nut crumble over the top (you can also mix it in a bit, if you want).

Bake for 25 to 35 minutes or until the squash is tender. Remove from the oven and serve bubbly and hot.

YIELD: 4 to 6 servings

SERVING SUGGESTIONS AND VARIATIONS

- Serve as a side or even over a small grain, such as quinoa or millet. Because the squash and tomatoes break down from the heat in the oven, they form a bit of a thin sauce that is delicious (infused with the cheesy pine nuts and garlic!).
- Sun Gold tomatoes, my favorite for this recipe and in general, are a very sweet variety of cherry tomatoes we grow in our garden every year.

PER SERVING: 125 Calories; 10g Fat (63.6% calories from fat); 3g Protein; 9g Carbohydrate; 3g Dietary Fiber; 0mg Cholesterol; 7mg Sodium

South African Yellow Rice (*Geelrys*)

▶ *Wheat-free, oil-free, soy-free if using soy-free Earth Balance*

Geelrys, one of many South African dishes with roots in the Dutch East Indies, sparkles with bright yellow color. The name *geelrys* literally means "yellow rice."

6 cups (1410 ml) water

2 cups (370 g) long-grain brown rice

1 tablespoon (13 g) granulated sugar

½ teaspoon turmeric

1 tablespoon (18 g) salt

2 tablespoons (28 g) nondairy butter
  (such as Earth Balance)

1 cinnamon stick

1 cup (145 g) raisins

Zest from 1 lemon

compassionate cooks' tip

To prevent the rice from turning out sticky after it's cooked, try this trick. Once your rice is cooked to the desired texture, turn off the heat, and leave it covered for 10 minutes. Then, lift up the cover and fluff. It works every time.

DIRECTIONS

In a 3-quart (3 L) saucepan, bring the water to a boil. Add the rice, sugar, turmeric, salt, butter, cinnamon stick, raisins, and lemon zest. Stir to combine.

Cover and simmer for 35 to 45 minutes over medium heat until the rice is cooked.

Remove the cinnamon stick and fluff with a fork.

YIELD: 7 cups (1155 g)

SERVING SUGGESTION AND VARIATIONS

- Spoon the bright yellow rice into a pretty serving bowl in a contrasting color, such as red or green. Place a couple of cinnamon sticks on top of the rice.
- *Geelrys* is a great accompaniment to casserole-style dishes, such as the Cajun Okra on page 121 or the Southern-Style Succotash on page 237.

PER SERVING: 149 Calories; 2g Fat (13.8% calories from fat); 2g Protein; 30g Carbohydrate; 2g Dietary Fiber; 0mg Cholesterol; 505mg Sodium

Hot Tamale Pie

▶ *Wheat-free, oil-free, soy-free if using soy-free Earth Balance*

This irresistible tamale pie is made with beans, lots of vegetables and spices, and a crust of cornmeal. It keeps well in the refrigerator for up to 5 days.

1 tablespoon (15 ml) water, for sautéing

1 medium red onion, finely chopped

2 bell peppers (yellow, red, orange, or green), seeded and chopped

2 cloves garlic, minced

3½ cups (825 ml) water, divided

3 medium tomatoes, seeded and chopped

1 can (15 ounces, or 420 g) pinto beans, rinsed and drained

1 can (15 ounces, or 420 g) kidney beans, rinsed and drained

1 can (15 ounces, or 420 g) black beans, rinsed and drained

1½ cups corn (315 g canned, 246 g frozen, or 231 g fresh)

2 tablespoons (12 g) chili powder

1 teaspoon ground cumin

¼ teaspoon cayenne pepper

1 teaspoon salt, or as needed, divided

3 cups (705 ml) water

1 cup (140 g) coarse cornmeal

1 tablespoon (15 ml) freshly squeezed lemon juice

¼ cup (24 g) nutritional yeast flakes (optional)

DIRECTIONS

Preheat the oven to 325°F (170°C, or gas mark 3).

Heat the water in a large sauté pan over medium-high heat. Add the onion, bell peppers, and garlic and cook until softened, 5 to 7 minutes. Stir in ½ cup (120 ml) of the water, tomatoes, beans, corn, chili powder, cumin, cayenne, and ½ teaspoon of the salt.

Cover and cook for 10 to 15 minutes until the vegetables soften and the flavors meld. Pour into a 9 x 13-inch (23 x 33 cm) baking dish.

Meanwhile, in a 3-quart (3 L) saucepan, bring the remaining 3 cups (705 ml) water to a boil. Add the cornmeal and remaining ½ teaspoon salt and whisk to combine. Return to a boil over medium-high heat and then immediately reduce the heat to low and simmer, stirring often, until thickened, about 5 minutes. Add the nutritional yeast and stir to combine. Taste for seasoning, adding more salt if necessary, and turn off the heat.

Spoon and spread the cooked cornmeal over the bean mixture. Use the back of a moistened wooden spoon to make spreading easier.

Bake for 30 minutes or until the mixture is hot and bubbling. Cool for 10 minutes before serving.

YIELD: 8 servings

SERVING SUGGESTIONS AND VARIATIONS

I recommend adding some chipotle chile powder for a bit of a smoky kick!

PER SERVING: 263 Calories; 4g Fat (11.9% calories from fat); 13g Protein; 47g Carbohydrate; 12g Dietary Fiber; 0mg Cholesterol; 857mg Sodium

food lore

A traditional Mexican dish, tamales comprise a sweet or savory corn mixture wrapped in corn-husks and steamed. This version retains the flavor of the original but modifies the form.

advance preparation required

Swiss Chard Pie

▶ *Wheat-free*

This crustless custard-like pie is perfect for brunch, lunch, or dinner and cuts some calories by leaving out the pastry. For a more decadent version, however, you can certainly use a store-bought pie crust or phyllo pastry.

1 tablespoon (15 ml) oil or water, for sautéing

1 medium yellow onion, chopped

2 cloves garlic, minced

1 bunch Swiss chard (red, yellow, white, or rainbow), chopped into bite-size pieces

¾ teaspoon salt, plus more to taste, divided

12 ounces (340 g) extra-firm tofu

¼ teaspoon turmeric

¼ teaspoon nutmeg

¼ teaspoon cayenne pepper

¾ cup Cashew Cheese (page 78)

1 tablespoon (2.5 g) minced fresh basil

Freshly ground pepper, to taste

PER SERVING: 183 Calories; 14g Fat (65.7% calories from fat); 7g Protein; 9g Carbohydrate; 2g Dietary Fiber; 0mg Cholesterol; 406mg Sodium

DIRECTIONS

Preheat the oven to 375°F (190°C, or gas mark 5). Spray a 9-inch (23 cm) ceramic pie pan lightly with nonstick spray.

In a large sauté pan heat the oil, and sauté the onion and garlic until the onion is translucent, about 5 minutes.

Add the chard to the pan, reduce the heat, and cover until all the chard is wilted. Season to taste with salt and remove from the heat. Drain any extra water that may have accumulated.

Place the tofu, the remaining ¾ teaspoon salt, turmeric, nutmeg, and cayenne pepper in a blender and purée until smooth. Transfer to a large bowl and stir in the cooked chard, cashew cheese, and basil. Taste and season as necessary, adding a little more cashew cheese, salt, or spices, as desired.

Combine thoroughly and pour into the prepared pie pan.

Bake for 40 to 45 minutes or until the center is set and the top is a beautiful golden brown. Remove from the oven and allow to rest for 30 minutes before slicing and serving.

YIELD: 4 to 6 servings

SERVING SUGGESTIONS AND VARIATIONS

Other greens, especially spinach, can substitute for the chard.

compassionate cooks' tips

• Although the leaves are the tenderest part of the chard plant, you can certainly eat the stems and ribs as well. Just chop them up small so they're finished cooking at the same time as the leaves.

• The amount of Cashew Cheese you'll use for this will leave you with enough left over to combine it with macaroni for a delicious macaroni and cheese.

EAT FOOD, NOT PILLS

Recently, there has been more and more evidence of the healing power of antioxidants—particularly beta-carotene, vitamin A, vitamin E, vitamin C, selenium, and zinc—and as a result, they have been isolated and sold as pills.

Living as we do in a quick-fix, pill-popping society, we are tempted to believe that all the healthful properties of food can be whittled down into a single magic pill to act as a panacea to counter our poor lifestyle habits.

Let me try and break this to you gently: there is no magic pill!

Not only is that the wrong way to approach healthful living, but it is also not possible. Intelligent though we are and sophisticated though our science is, nature's complexity wins every time.

The truth is, we have no business trying to extract out a single beneficial element from plants. It just doesn't work that way. All of the factors that make up a plant—the phytochemicals, the fiber, and the vitamins within—all work together to create the benefit we receive. The nutrients found in plants come perfectly packaged.

Also, when we eat a certain food, we're not getting just *one* phytochemical or *one* vitamin. Some foods may contain up to 100 compounds, so we're simply not getting the true benefits just from taking a pill.

What's more, recent research does suggest that taking certain antioxidant supplements might actually be harmful. Neither the scientific community nor the government sets an upper limit for the consumption of antioxidants *from food*, but there is concern about getting antioxidants in a pill. (See "Are Antioxidant Supplements Safe?" on pages 86 and 87.)

That is not to say that some people don't need supplements in certain situations, but most of us can do a better job turning to nature rather than a pill.

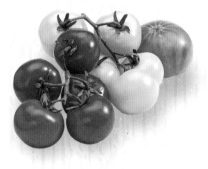

Cornmeal Blueberry Porridge (*Sautauthig*)

▶ *Wheat-free, soy-free depending on the milk used, oil-free*

Pronounced SAW-taw-teeg, this was a favorite dish of the eastern Native American tribes. Originally, it was a simple pudding made with crushed blueberries and dried cracked corn; later, the European settlers added milk, butter, and sugar when they were available.

3 cups (705 ml) water, plus more for drizzling

1½ cups (353 ml) nondairy milk (such as almond, soy, rice, hazelnut, hemp, or oat)

1½ cups (210 g) coarse cornmeal (also called polenta)

½ teaspoon salt, or to taste

3 tablespoons (60 g) real maple syrup, plus more for drizzling

2 cups (300 g) fresh or (310 g) frozen blueberries

DIRECTIONS

In a 3-quart (3 L) saucepan, heat the water and milk until bubbles form around the edge of the pot.

Stirring constantly, slowly add the cornmeal and salt to taste. Stir to combine thoroughly and reduce the heat to low. Simmer for 5 to 10 minutes longer until thickened, stirring all the while.

Add the maple syrup, and stir to combine. Gently stir in the blueberries using a rubber spatula and turn off the heat. Serve in bowls, drizzled with a little additional maple syrup and milk.

YIELD: 6 to 8 servings

PER SERVING: 143 Calories; 1g Fat (7.5% calories from fat); 4g Protein; 30g Carbohydrate; 4g Dietary Fiber; 0mg Cholesterol; 144mg Sodium

food lore

In a letter to friends back in England, one colonist describes how sautauthig was prepared:

". . . this is to be boyled or stued with a gentle fire, till it be tender, of a fitt consistence, as of Rice so boyled, into which Milke, or butter be put either with sugar or without it, it is a food very pleasant . . . but it must be observed that it be very well boyled, the longer the better, some will let it be stuing the whole day: after it is Cold it groweth thicker, and is commonly Eaten by mixing a good Quantity of Milke amongst it."

compassionate cooks' tip

If using frozen berries, thaw them before adding, and keep in mind that the juice from the frozen berries may turn this dish a beautiful blue.

advance preparation required

Mango Saffron Mousse

▶ *Oil-free, wheat-freee*

This delicious mousse takes 5 minutes to put together, especially if you are using frozen mangoes. Saffron and mango blend beautifully together, not only in terms of flavor but also in terms of color.

1 bag (10 ounces, or 280 g) frozen mangoes (or 1 small mango, cubed), thawed
1 box (12 ounces, or 340 g) organic silken tofu, firm or extra-firm (Mori-Nu is a common brand)
¼ cup (50 g) granulated sugar
3 drops saffron extract

DIRECTIONS

Add the mangoes, tofu, sugar, and saffron to a blender or food processor. Blend until smooth. Transfer to a container and refrigerate for a minimum of 1 hour. This helps it set up but also provides the characteristic chill of a good mousse.

YIELD: 3 cups (670 g)

SERVING SUGGESTIONS AND VARIATIONS

• Top with a mixture of finely chopped fresh, seasonal fruit (such as pomegranate seeds, apples, or grapes), golden raisins, and chopped pistachios.
• The flesh of mangoes can have a bit of a fibrous texture to them, so use a good blender to purée them as much as possible.

PER SERVING: 89 Calories; 2g Fat (20.3% calories from fat); 4g Protein; 15g Carbohydrate; 1g Dietary Fiber; 0mg Cholesterol; 5mg Sodium

did you know?

Crocin, a carotenoid found in the crocus flower where saffron is derived, is responsible for the characteristic color of saffron and is considered a powerful antioxidant with anticancer and antidepressant properties.

compassionate cooks' tips

• Although it can be confusing to see "firm" on a box of *silken* tofu, there are degrees of texture even in this creamy food. The tofu you will be using for this is indeed silken but one that is designated as "firm" or "extra-firm."

• I recently discovered saffron extract, which works beautifully in a dessert like this and costs a fraction of saffron threads. See Resources and Recommendations.

did you know?

One mango provides 160 percent of the Daily Value of vitamin A and 95 percent of the Daily Value of vitamin C!

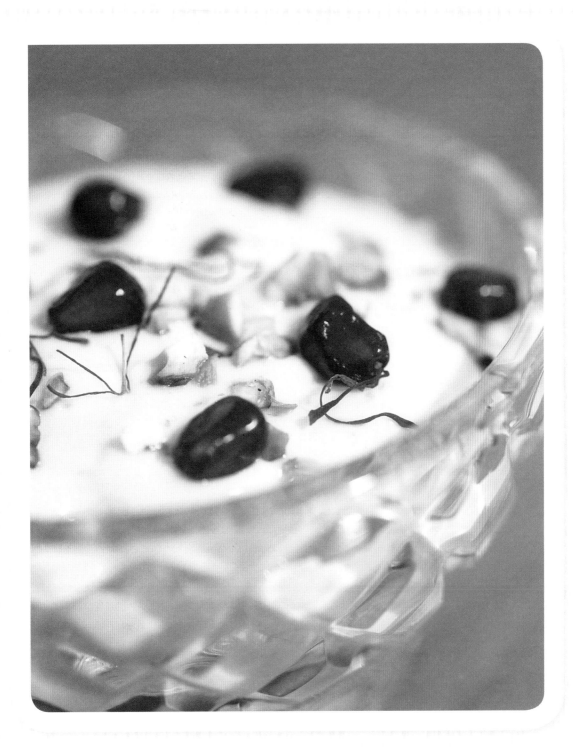

advance preparation required

Pineapple and Bananas with Ginger Syrup

▶ *Wheat-free, oil-free, soy-free*

This is a refreshing dessert that can be put together in minutes, especially once you have the syrup prepared and in the fridge.

1 cup (235 ml) water
¼ cup (80 g) agave nectar
¼ cup (25 g) peeled and minced or
    thinly sliced fresh ginger
1 medium pineapple, peeled, cored, and
    cut into 1-inch (2.5 cm) chunks
4 ripe bananas, sliced
Mint leaves, for garnish

PER SERVING: 263 Calories; 1g Fat (4.5% calories from fat); 2g Protein; 67g Carbohydrate; 6g Dietary Fiber; 0mg Cholesterol; 6mg Sodium

DIRECTIONS

Add the water, agave nectar, and ginger to a medium saucepan and cook over medium heat until the ingredients reduce and become somewhat syrupy. Strain and refrigerate for at least 1 hour, giving the syrup a chance to thicken slightly and chill.

When ready to serve, combine the pineapple and bananas in a medium bowl, transfer to serving bowls, and drizzle with the ginger syrup. Garnish with mint leaves and serve.

YIELD: 4 servings

SERVING SUGGESTIONS AND VARIATIONS

The ginger syrup pairs well with any fruit, so use your imagination and whatever you have on hand or in your garden.

compassionate cooks' tip

Because the banana wouldn't hold up well in the fridge once it's already cut, I would wait until the last minute to peel and slice. The pineapple, however, can be cut in advance and stored in the refrigerator.

advance preparation required

Frozen Banana Dessert

▶ *Soy-free depending on the milk used, wheat-free, oil-free*

Although we tend to think of decadent sugar-laden concoctions when we think of ice cream, I want to offer this alternative. One of the satisfying aspects of ice cream is its creamy texture, and this recipe has it in spades—with no added fat, sugar, or dairy! You will find me eating this several times a week.

2 ripe bananas, peeled and broken into chunks

2 Medjool dates (or other type of date), pitted

¼ cup (60 ml) nondairy milk (such as almond, soy, rice, hazelnut, hemp, or oat), or as much as needed to reach desired consistency

2 to 3 tablespoons (30 to 45 ml) orange or pineapple juice (optional)

Dash of ground cinnamon

PER SERVING: 152 Calories; 1g Fat (6.6% calories from fat); 2g Protein; 37g Carbohydrate; 4g Dietary Fiber; 0mg Cholesterol; 5mg Sodium

compassionate cooks' tip

Although this can be done in a regular blender, I confess the Vitamix (a super-high-powered blender) does the job better than any other.

DIRECTIONS

Freeze the banana chunks for several hours. (Personally, I always have a stash of frozen bananas in my freezer. I buy super-ripe bananas from the grocery when they're on sale, peel them all, break them up, and store them in plastic bags in the freezer. They're perfect for breakfast smoothies or for this type of treat.)

Add the frozen bananas and dates to a high-speed blender. Slowly add the milk and juice while you purée the bananas. You may need to turn off the blender and pull them away from the blade with a fork a few times. Continue this process until you have a creamy consistency. Add a dash of cinnamon at the end of processing.

Transfer to 2 serving bowls and sprinkle with a little more cinnamon.

YIELD: 2 servings

SERVING SUGGESTIONS AND VARIATIONS

Top with chopped nuts, such as walnuts, pecans, or peanuts.

WAYS TO INCREASE YELLOW FOODS

- Add lemon zest or lemon slices to main dishes, side dishes, or salads.

- Make fresh lemonade and add lemon peels to the pitcher before serving.

- Use spaghetti squash in place of wheat-based pasta. Top with your favorite pasta sauce.

- Make a tropical yellow fruit salad with mangoes, bananas, and pineapples.

- Choose yellow bell pepper when making a stir-fry or add it to salads or eat it as a snack with hummus.

- Grill or roast yellow bell peppers.

- Dice yellow bell peppers and sprinkle them on top of a homemade pizza.

- Drink natural lemonade, pineapple juice, or mango juice.

- Serve fresh chunks of pineapple, slices of bananas, and sliced yellow-skinned apples with peanut butter.

- Add pineapple chunks to your pizza.

- Mash rutabagas instead of or along with your mashed yellow potatoes.

- Choose yellow beets instead of red.

- Add yellow gooseberries to your salad.

- Vary watermelon by choosing yellow as well as red.

- Add edible yellow flowers to salad, including nasturtiums, dandelions, and honeysuckle.

- Use yellow tomatoes in place of red in the Gazpacho recipe (page 23).

- Peel overripe bananas and freeze to use in fruit smoothies.

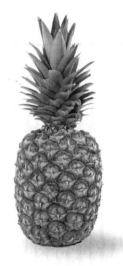

Caramelized Bananas

▶ *Wheat-free, oil-free, soy-free if using soy-free Earth Balance*

Cooking bananas (whether you're baking, grilling, sautéing, or broiling) brings out their natural sugar, making this favorite fruit of mine even more delectable than when it's raw.

4 ripe bananas

2 to 3 tablespoons (30 to 45 g) light brown sugar, or to taste

2 tablespoons (26 g) granulated sugar

½ teaspoon ground cinnamon, or to taste

2 tablespoons (28 g) nondairy butter (such as Earth Balance)

DIRECTIONS

Preheat the oven to 350°F (180°C, or gas mark 4). Lightly grease a piece of parchment paper using non-dairy butter and place on a baking sheet.

Peel the bananas and halve lengthwise. Place on the prepared baking sheet, cut side up.

In a bowl, combine the brown sugar, granulated sugar, and cinnamon and sprinkle over the bananas. Dot with the butter.

Bake for 25 minutes or until golden brown and caramelized. Serve hot or at room temperature.

YIELD: 4 servings

SERVING SUGGESTIONS AND VARIATIONS

Serve with nondairy ice cream, nondairy yogurt, or Avocado Pudding (page 128).

PER SERVING: 116 Calories; 5g Fat (39.9% calories from fat); trace Protein; 18g Carbohydrate; trace Dietary Fiber; 0mg Cholesterol; 5mg Sodium

did you know?

Most of us correctly associate bananas with potassium, but few know the role of this essential mineral. Best known as a blood pressure regulator, potassium protects against heart disease, hypoglycemia, diabetes, and kidney disease. Helping to keep muscles strong, it also eliminates irritability, confusion, and stress. Potassium is also a natural diuretic, which means it causes the body to excrete both water and sodium. In fact, many experts agree that high blood pressure is caused as much by low potassium as by high sodium. Other potassium-rich foods include lima beans, papayas, plantains, pears, mangoes, cantaloupe, cucumbers, tomatoes, and oat bran.

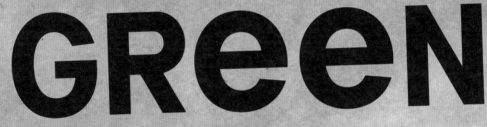

color me
GREEN

THE PIGMENT OF LIFE

MOST OF OUR ASSOCIATIONS with the color green are positive (we'll just ignore Shakespeare's *green with envy* coinage for now), and I'm not just referring to the *green stuff* (you know: the cashish, the moolah, the dough, the bread). Talented gardeners have a *green thumb*. Approved actions get the *green light*. To have the *rub of the green* is to have good luck, and to *live a green lifestyle* means to tread lightly on our vulnerable planet. (We can talk about "green-washing" another time.)

When it comes to the nutrient density of foods, green vegetables win *every time*. Think about which vegetables we all need to "eat more of." Broccoli, Brussels sprouts, asparagus, spinach, kale, collard greens, green beans, lima beans, and peas most likely come to mind rather effortlessly. Green is literally the color of life.

This is all because of a pigment called chlorophyll. In fact, chlorophyll is the most abundant plant pigment in nature. Chlorophyll (from the Greek *chloros*, meaning "green," and *phyllon*, meaning "leaf") provides the green color found in grasses, leaves, and many of the vegetables we eat. We don't tend to think of chlorophyll playing a role in our health, but it is, in fact, vital. After all, chlorophyll is vital to photosynthesis, a process that allows plants to obtain energy from light. Through photosynthesis, plants convert carbon dioxide and water into carbohydrates and release oxygen into the atmosphere. Without carbohydrates (the main fuel of the brain) and oxygen (life's force), we would be in a pretty sorry state.

When You "Eat Green," You "Eat a Rainbow"

Although it is true that the more colors we eat, the more nutrients we consume, when it comes to green, we are actually eating a variety of different colors. When we eat green leafy vegetables, we eat *all* colors.

To fully absorb this, think about what happens to leaves in the autumn when they change from green to yellow or orange or red. These colors are actually in the leaves year-round, but they get overshadowed by the green color, which is the chlorophyll in the leaves. (The same goes for a green banana or tomato whose chlorophyll disappears when it ripens to unmask its yellow or red skin.) So, when you consume green leafy vegetables (particularly kale, spinach, collard greens, Swiss chard, beet greens, arugula, romaine, watercress, and bok choy), you're actually eating a variety of colors—and thus, a variety of phytonutrients and antioxidants, such as beta-carotene and lutein.

In fact, the reason plants make carotenoids like lutein and beta-carotene, which are powerful antioxidants (see page 45 for a further explanation), is to protect themselves against the free radicals that are generated when sunlight strikes chlorophyll. The darker the green vegetable, the more chlorophyll it contains and the greater its need for antioxidant protection. Those antioxidants exist to protect the plant's cells; in turn, when we consume them, they protect our cells.

Green Sources

Our green chapter features a variety of green plant foods—and not just veggies! Among the artichokes, asparagus, broccoli rabe, Brussels sprouts, celery, cabbage, collard greens, cucumbers, edamame, fennel, green onions, green beans, green bell peppers, jalapeño peppers, kale, limes, lettuce, okra, peas, spinach, Swiss chard, and zucchini squash, you will find such fruits as avocado, cucumbers, green grapes, honeydew, and kiwi; nuts such as pistachios; and seeds such as pumpkin.

Not only that, but fresh herbs factor in a great deal, including basil, cilantro, parsley, sage, thyme, oregano, marjoram, and mint—adding color, flavor, and nutrition.

Those green plant foods not found in this chapter may be found in other chapters as minor players or complementing other colors in the rainbow chapter.

Personally, I aspire to consume a pound of greens every day—every single day—and that's really not that hard if you center your diet on whole plant foods. Even if you don't reach that goal, just by trying to attain it, you will substantially increase your consumption of the green stuff.

ADVANCE PREPARATION REQUIRED

Asian-Inspired Edamame Salad

▶ *Wheat-free*

A quick, convenient, light meal, snack, or side dish, this is one of my go-to favorites any time of the year.

8 cups (1880 ml) water

1 tablespoon (18 g) salt

1 pound (455 g) frozen, shelled edamame

¼ cup (60 ml) seasoned or plain rice vinegar

1 tablespoon (15 ml) toasted sesame oil

1 tablespoon (15 ml) tamari soy sauce

1 tablespoon (20 g) agave nectar

1 teaspoon lemon juice

1 teaspoon salt

½ teaspoon freshly ground pepper

2 carrots, shredded

2 tablespoons (16 g) sesame seeds (raw or toasted)

DIRECTIONS

Place the water and salt in a soup pot and bring to a boil. Add the edamame and cook for 5 minutes. Rinse immediately with cold water, drain well, and set aside.

Meanwhile, in a large bowl, whisk together the vinegar, oil, tamari, agave, lemon juice, salt, and pepper.

Add the drained edamame to the bowl, along with the carrots and sesame seeds. Toss well to combine. Chill for at least 2 hours or overnight.

Bring to room temperature 30 minutes before serving.

YIELD: 4 servings

PER SERVING: 274 Calories; 14g Fat (42.6% calories from fat); 17g Protein; 25g Carbohydrate; 7g Dietary Fiber; 0mg Cholesterol; 2385mg Sodium

food lore

In Japanese, edamame literally means "twig bean" (*eda* = "twig" + *mame* = "bean") in reference to the short stem at the end of the pod.

did you know?

Packing a substantial nutritional punch, just ½ cup (75 g) of shelled edamame beans yields 4 grams of fiber, 9 grams of protein, 8 percent of the Daily Value for vitamin C, and 10 percent of the Daily Value for iron.

Sweet Pea "Guacamole"

▶ *Oil-free, wheat-free, soy-free*

This is a simple, delicious, and fat-free variation of traditional guacamole. It has the added benefit of not turning brown like the avocado-based original.

1½ cups green peas, (225 g) fresh or
    (195 g) frozen (thawed)
1½ teaspoons ground cumin
½ yellow onion, coarsely chopped
2 or 3 large cloves garlic, peeled
2 to 3 tablespoons (30 to 45 ml) lemon
    juice, divided
¼ to ½ teaspoon crushed red pepper flakes
Salt and freshly ground pepper, to taste
1 or 2 fresh Roma or plum tomatoes,
    seeded and chopped
Cilantro, for garnish

DIRECTIONS

In a food processor or blender, combine the peas, cumin, onion, garlic, 2 tablespoons (30 ml) of the lemon juice, and red pepper flakes and blend until smooth. Taste, add salt, and adjust seasonings as necessary, adding more lemon juice if necessary and more red pepper flakes, if desired.

Blend for a few more seconds and then transfer to a serving bowl. Stir in the chopped tomatoes and garnish with cilantro. Serve with tortilla chips, crackers, or fresh veggies.

YIELD: 12 servings, about 2 tablespoons (30 g) each

PER SERVING: 24 Calories; trace Fat (7.1% calories from fat); 1g Protein; 5g Carbohydrate; 1g Dietary Fiber; 0mg Cholesterol; 4mg Sodium

did you know?

One cup (150 g) of green peas provides more than 50 percent of the Daily Value of vitamin K, which contributes to strong bones.

ADVANCE PREPARATION REQUIRED

Greek Spinach Salad

▶ *Wheat-free*

The thawed tofu here plays the role of the feta cheese usually called for in a Greek salad.

1 pound (455 g) spinach leaves, washed, rinsed, and patted dry

2 cucumbers, seeded and sliced (unpeeled)

1½ cups (200 g) crumbled thawed tofu (see below)

1 cup (100 g) kalamata olives, pitted and sliced

3 cups (540 g) diced Roma tomatoes

⅓ cup (37 g) chopped oil-packed sun-dried tomatoes, drained, oil reserved

½ red onion, sliced

2 to 3 tablespoons (30 to 45 ml) balsamic vinegar, to taste

½ teaspoon dried or 1 teaspoon fresh oregano

Salt and freshly ground pepper, to taste

DIRECTIONS

In a large bowl, toss together the spinach, cucumbers, crumbled tofu, olives, Roma tomatoes, sun-dried tomatoes, 2 tablespoons (30 ml) of the reserved sun-dried tomato oil, red onion, balsamic vinegar, and oregano. Season with a sprinkle of salt and a twist of the pepper mill.

Let the flavors mingle for 30 to 60 minutes before serving. Keep chilled until ready to serve.

YIELD: 8 servings

THAWED TOFU

Tofu can be frozen for up to 6 months. Thawed tofu has a pleasant caramel color and a chewy, spongy texture that soaks up marinade sauces and is great for the grill. (See page 181 for freezing and thawing tofu.)

PER SERVING: 143 Calories; 10g Fat (59.8% calories from fat); 5g Protein; 11g Carbohydrate; 3g Dietary Fiber; 0mg Cholesterol; 525mg Sodium

did you know?

Lutein, a carotenoid present in green vegetables such as spinach, kale, and broccoli, protects against age-related eye disease, such as macular degeneration and cataracts. Even though they contain significantly less lutein than does spinach, egg yolks are often touted as a good source of lutein, most likely due to the *fat* in the yolk. Lutein, like other carotenoids, is fat-soluble and cannot be absorbed unless fat is also present. To boost your lutein absorption from spinach, I suggest enjoying this leafy green along with a little fat, such as in this salad, which contains some good fat (in the tofu) and some oil (in the sun-dried tomatoes).

Walnut Basil Pesto

▶ *Wheat-free, soy-free, oil-free variation*

As with all pesto, this one can be modified to suit your taste. It is easy to prepare and rich in healthful fats, so make a large batch and freeze some for future use.

2 cups (80 g) loosely packed fresh basil leaves
⅓ cup (33 g) raw walnuts
2 or 3 cloves garlic
3 to 4 tablespoons (45 to 60 ml) olive oil
1 tablespoon (15 ml) lemon juice
½ teaspoon salt, or to taste

DIRECTIONS

Combine the basil, walnuts, and garlic in a food processor and blend until the ingredients are finely chopped, scraping down the sides of the bowl as necessary.

Add the oil slowly and a little at a time and process until smooth and creamy. (You don't need a lot of oil—just add enough to smooth it out a little.) Add the lemon juice and salt to taste.

YIELD: ¾ cup (195 g)

SERVING SUGGESTIONS AND VARIATIONS

- For an oil-free version, eliminate the oil and replace it with 1 to 2 tablespoons (16 to 32 g) light miso.
- Although you'll have to change the name of the recipe, you can replace the basil with parsley or cilantro and the walnuts with pine nuts.

PER SERVING: 124 Calories; 13g Fat (91.1% calories from fat); 1g Protein; 2g Carbohydrate; 1g Dietary Fiber; 0mg Cholesterol; 178mg Sodium

compassionate cooks' tip

Use purple basil instead of green and garnish the plate with some whole green and purple leaves for a dramatic effect. (Note: there is purple Italian basil and purple Thai basil. You won't want to use the latter for pesto.)

Edamame Soup

▶ *Wheat-free, oil-free if eliminating the oil garnish*

This beautiful olive-colored soup is surprisingly rich and creamy and made even tastier by the addition of toasted sesame oil drizzled on top just before serving.

1 tablespoon (15 ml) water, for sautéing

1 medium yellow onion, chopped

1 yellow potato, peeled and cubed

1 package (10 or 12 ounces, or 280 or 340 g) frozen edamame or lima beans, thawed

4 cups (940 ml) vegetable stock

Salt and freshly ground pepper, to taste

Toasted sesame oil, for garnish

compassionate cooks' tip

My high-powered blender purées the chunky ingredients into a silky smooth soup. If your blender or food processor doesn't create the creamy results you're looking for, try pressing it through a fine-mesh strainer.

DIRECTIONS

In a soup pot, heat the water over medium heat and add the chopped onion. Sauté for about 5 minutes until it turns translucent. Add the potato, edamame, and stock, cover, and cook until the potatoes are fork-tender, 20 to 25 minutes.

Transfer the soup to a blender or food processor (or use an immersion blender) and purée until smooth. Add salt and pepper to taste and purée again. Return the puréed soup to the pot and reheat gently without boiling.

Ladle into bowls, drizzle a small amount of toasted sesame oil on top, and serve hot.

YIELD: 6 servings

SERVING SUGGESTIONS AND VARIATIONS

In addition to or instead of the sesame oil, add lightly fried scallions, crushed toasted peanuts, a slight squeeze of lemon juice, or a dollop of nondairy sour cream to each serving bowl.

PER SERVING: 130 Calories; 5g Fat (31.8% calories from fat); 9g Protein; 15g Carbohydrate; 3g Dietary Fiber; 0mg Cholesterol; 673mg Sodium

BEING GREEN

Calorie for calorie, dark green leafy vegetables are perhaps the most concentrated source of nutrients of any food. They are a rich source of minerals (including iron, calcium, potassium, and magnesium) and vitamins, including vitamins K, C, E, and many of the B vitamins. They also provide a variety of phytonutrients, including beta-carotene and lutein, which protect our cells from damage and our eyes from age-related problems. Great sources of fiber and folate, they're low in fat, high in protein per calorie, and even contain small amounts of omega-3 fats.

Technically, there are more than 1,000 species of plants with edible leaves, and I clearly can't cover them all here. With so many plants with edibles leaves, I'm flabbergasted when people say, "Being vegan seems so limiting!" Just in terms of green leafy vegetables, we're talking more than 1,000 plant species.

The evidence of the healthfulness of greens is overwhelming. Countless human-based studies and research support our need to consume lots of green leafies. Research shows they protect our bodies against heart disease and a number of different cancers, strengthen our immune system, protect our bones against degeneration, promote lung health, lower cholesterol, enhance our mental performance, lower our risk for cataracts, protect against rheumatoid arthritis, help the colon function properly, act as anti-inflammatories, and provide energy—just name it.

Although tips, information, and food lore abound throughout this cookbook, I thought I would elaborate on some of the better-known green leafies. Most greens are interchangeable in recipes, so be creative and adventurous!

Arugula, eaten in ancient Rome, is also known as rocket arugula and rocket greens. It has a peppery flavor and can be eaten raw in salads or added to stir-fries, soups, and pasta sauces. It's pretty powerful on its own, so it's often mixed with milder greens to lessen the bitter flavor. It can also be sautéed in olive oil, like most greens, and if you really don't like it, most any green can be substituted for it, the closest matches being Belgian endive, escarole, and dandelion greens. Try arugula pesto using arugula instead of basil.

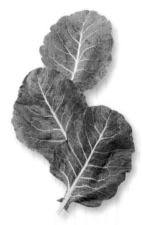

Collard greens date back to prehistoric times. With a spinach-like flavor, collards are actually a member of the cabbage family and are thus closely related to kale. In fact, the ancient Greeks grew kale and collards and made no distinction between them. The traditional way to cook greens is to boil or simmer slowly with a piece of pig, but I recommend using smoked peppers (chipotles) or liquid smoke to get the same effect without harming anyone. The salt and smokiness adds flavor but also tempers the tough texture of the collard greens and softens what some think is a bitter flavor. Cook the greens until they are very soft and serve with freshly baked cornbread.

Dandelion greens are a perennial (i.e. relentless) lawn weed in much of the northern hemisphere, but they are also a nutritious addition to your diet. Dandelion greens are available in stores and at farmers' markets, but feel free to harvest the greens that grow around your house. DO NOT eat them if your lawn is chemically treated. Eaten raw, they are wonderful tossed into salads, where they add a peppery spiciness. Lightly boiled, sprinkled with salt and a bit of cider vinegar, they are an easy and delicious side dish. Alternatively, you can sauté them with a little garlic, olive oil, red pepper flakes, and some salt, and you're good to go. (The stems may be bitter, so stick with the leaves.)

Kale is a member of the cabbage family, like broccoli, cauliflower, and Brussels sprouts, and it's incredibly nutritious. It is my favorite green leafy. There are a lot of different kinds of kale. Black Palm kale, also known as Lacinato, dinosaur kale, or Nero Di Toscana, is the favored variety grown in Italy. Other popular kale varieties include Red Russian, Siberian, Red Ursa, White Russian, Dwarf Blue Curled Scotch, Konserva, Redbor, Winterbor, Premier, Hanover Salad, and Starbor.

Mustard greens have a hot, spicy flavor, and, like kale, they have an obscene amount of vitamin K; they have lots of vitamin A and C, lots of folate, lots of fiber, and a good amount of protein, with 3 grams of protein in 1 cup (140 g) of cooked mustard greens. There are a variety of mustard greens as well, but for our purposes, I'm talking about what is called Southern mustard or American mustard greens. They're sold as mature greens and look like a delicate version of kale, having jade green leaves that are crinkled or ruffled but are more tender than kale. And yes, mustard—the condiment—comes from mustard the plant, which produces the brown seeds used to make Dijon mustard.

(continued on next page)

(continued from previous page)

Spinach is what most people think of first and foremost when they think of a green leafy vegetable. A green on the sweeter side, it's also rich in vitamins K, A, and C, iron, and phytochemicals. My favorite way to eat spinach is raw and in a salad, tossed with some balsamic vinaigrette, toasted pecans, and cranberries (in the fall) or raspberries (in the summer). As with most greens, spinach will shrink substantially, so when a recipe calls for a cup or two (30 to 60 g) of raw spinach, and it seems to overflow and not fit in the pan, give it a few minutes. When it cooks, it shrinks—a lot.

Swiss chard, along with kale, is one of my favorite greens, which I grow and eat in abundance! Chard belongs to the same family as beets and spinach and is similar in taste: it has the bitterness of beet greens and the slightly salty flavor of spinach leaves. Both the leaves and the stalks are edible, although the stems vary in texture, with the white ones being the most tender. Chard is also packed with vitamins K, A, and C and has lots of vitamin E, fiber, folate, calcium, iron, and potassium.

Cleaning Greens

One of the best ways to clean greens is by dunking them in a bowl of water and then rinsing. Be sure to wash only if you are going to prepare the greens right away. They tend to be highly perishable and should not be stored wet. Store unwashed greens wrapped in a plastic bag in the refrigerator for up to 3 days.

May you find abundance in the 1,000 edible leaves available to us, health in their healing properties, and solace in the awareness that no animal need be killed so that we may live.

Spinach Soup with Basil and Dill

▶ *Oil-free, wheat-free*

The color of this complex-tasting soup will make you leap with joy.

3 medium yellow potatoes, peeled and cubed

2 medium yellow onions, chopped

5 cloves garlic, minced

6 cups (1410 ml) vegetable stock

1 teaspoon salt (or more, to taste)

1½ pounds (683 g) fresh spinach, cleaned and coarsely chopped

½ cup (32 g) minced fresh dill

8 fresh basil leaves, minced

½ cup (120 ml) nondairy milk (such as almond, soy, rice, hemp, hazelnut, or oat)

2 to 3 tablespoons (40 to 60 g) agave nectar

Juice from 1 fresh lemon, divided

Freshly ground pepper, to taste

Nondairy sour cream, for topping

DIRECTIONS

Add the potatoes, onions, garlic, stock, and salt to a large soup pot. Bring to a boil and then cover and simmer very slowly for about 20 minutes or until the potatoes can be pierced with a fork.

Use a food processor or blender to purée the soup, adding the spinach, dill, and basil. You may need to do this in more than one batch, scraping down the sides of the bowl or pitcher, as necessary.

Return the puréed soup to the pot and add the milk, agave nectar, and juice from ½ a lemon. Taste and add more lemon, if necessary. Increase the heat (but not to boiling), season with salt and pepper as needed, and serve hot with a dollop of nondairy sour cream.

YIELD: 4 servings

SERVING SUGGESTIONS AND VARIATIONS

Any of the following toppings would be great additions: finely minced apple, toasted pumpkin seeds, or pomegranate seeds.

PER SERVING: 249 Calories; 3g Fat (9.3% calories from fat); 9g Protein; 53g Carbohydrate; 9g Dietary Fiber; 0mg Cholesterol; 2169mg Sodium

did you know?

When you think of spinach, who do you think of? Popeye, of course! So strong, muscular, and energetic was Popeye. His counterpart, of course, was Wimpy—literally—and his staple food was hamburgers. I can't help believing that Popeye's creator knew a little something about nutrition because, in fact, spinach is an excellent source of iron, a mineral that is abundant in plant foods from lentils and beans to green leafy vegetables. One cup of steamed spinach provides 35.7 percent of the Daily Value for iron, whose absorption is increased in the presence of vitamin C. In this soup, you'll find it in the lemon juice.

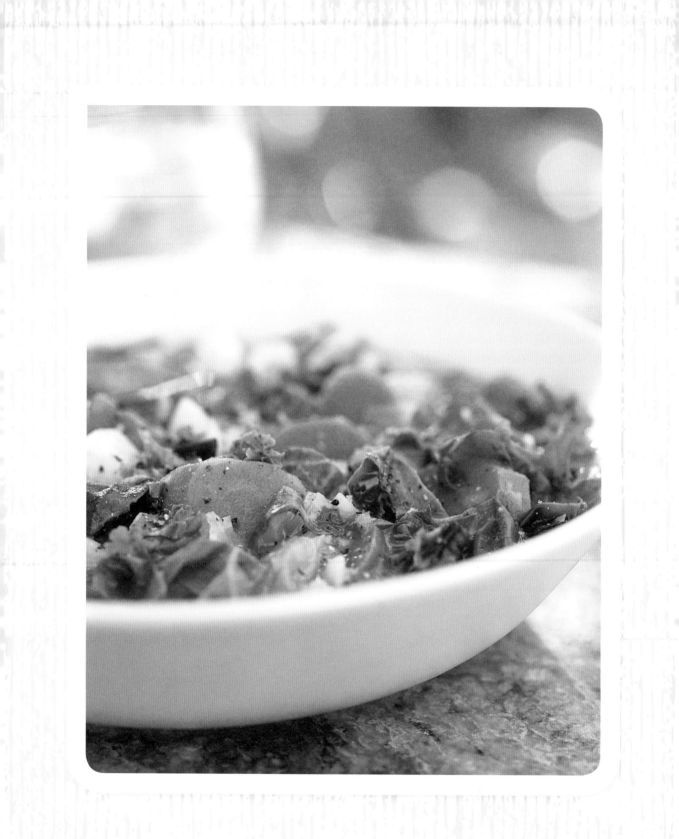

Three-Greens Ribollita Soup

▶ *Soy-free, oil-free if using water for sautéing, wheat-free if eliminating the bread*

Ribollita means "twice-cooked," or "reboiled," in Italian. A white bean stock is livened up with greens, carrots, and potatoes, with added slices of toasted bread.

2 cans (15 ounces, or 420 g) cannellini
    beans, drained and rinsed

4 cups (940 ml) vegetable stock

5 cloves garlic, minced

4 fresh sage leaves

2 bay leaves

½ teaspoon salt

2 tablespoons (30 ml) oil or water, for sautéing

2 medium yellow onions, diced

3 carrots, coarsely chopped

2 potatoes, peeled and diced

½ cup (45 g) coarsely chopped cabbage

1 bunch Swiss chard, trimmed and chopped
    into bite-size pieces

1 bunch kale, trimmed and chopped into
    bite-size pieces

2 cups (470 ml) water or vegetable stock

Salt and freshly ground black pepper, to taste

6 or 12 (½ inch, or 1.3 cm, thick) slices hearty
    Italian or French bread, lightly toasted

DIRECTIONS

Place the beans, vegetable stock, garlic, sage leaves, bay leaves, and salt in a saucepan. Simmer over low-medium heat until the mixture begins to thicken and the flavor of the garlic and herbs begin to infuse the beans, about 20 minutes. (You may also purée the beans first and then add to pot.)

Discard the bay and sage leaves. Transfer to a blender or food processor and blend until smooth. Set aside. (If you purée the beans first, you can skip this step.)

In a large soup pot, heat the oil over medium-high heat. Add the onions; cook and stir until translucent, about 7 minutes. Add the carrots, potatoes, cabbage, Swiss chard, kale, the puréed bean mixture, and the water. Season with salt and pepper to taste. Cover and cook until the potatoes are fork-tender, about 20 minutes, stirring at least once.

Adjust the seasonings to taste. At this point you can either serve it right away or refrigerate it overnight and reboil the next day.

When ready to serve, place 1 or 2 toasted bread slices in the bottom of each serving bowl and ladle the soup over the bread. Serve.

YIELD: 6 servings

SERVING SUGGESTIONS AND VARIATIONS

To add a delicious tomato flavor and beautiful red color to the soup, replace 1 cup (235 ml) of the 2 cups (470 ml) water with 1 cup (235 ml) tomato juice, or add 1 tablespoon (16 g) tomato paste when you add the 2 cups (470 ml) water.

PER SERVING: 434 Calories; 7g Fat (14.9% calories from fat); 21g Protein; 74g Carbohydrate; 14g Dietary Fiber; 0mg Cholesterol; 1346mg Sodium

food lore

Swiss chard is not native to Switzerland; a Swiss botanist determined the scientific name of this plant in the nineteenth century, and since then its name has honored his homeland. Chard actually originates in the Mediterranean region and got its common name from cardoon, a celery-like plant with thick stalks that resemble those of chard.

Summer Squash Soup

▷ *Oil-free if sautéing in water, wheat-free, soy-free*

This is a great soup to make when you have an abundance of summer squash from your garden or farmers' market.

1 tablespoon (15 ml) oil or water, for sautéing

1 large onion, chopped

3 cloves garlic, minced

1½ pounds (683 g) summer squash, chopped and unpeeled (2 medium)

1 jalapeño pepper, seeds and ribs removed and chopped

2 stalks celery, chopped

2 medium yellow potatoes, peeled and diced

4 cups (940 ml) vegetable stock

1 teaspoon dried oregano

1 teaspoon dried tarragon

2 teaspoons tahini (sesame seed paste)

Salt and white pepper, to taste

DIRECTIONS

Add the oil to a soup pot and heat over medium heat. Add the onion and cook for about 5 minutes until it begins to turn translucent. Add the garlic, squash, jalapeño pepper, and celery and sauté for 5 minutes longer or until all the vegetables start to sweat a bit.

Add the potatoes, stock, oregano, and tarragon, cover, and cook over medium heat until the potatoes are completely tender and able to be pierced with a fork, 20 to 25 minutes.

Transfer the soup to a blender or food processor (or use an immersion blender), along with the tahini and salt and pepper, and purée at high speed until completely smooth and creamy. Work in several batches if your blender is on the smaller side.

Return the soup to the pot and keep on low heat until ready to serve. Ladle into bowls and serve with a seasonal salad and hearty bread.

YIELD: 4 to 6 servings

PER SERVING: 115 Calories; 4g Fat (30.2% calories from fat); 3g Protein; 19g Carbohydrate; 4g Dietary Fiber; 0mg Cholesterol; 679mg Sodium

did you know?

Some people use white pepper in place of black pepper when they want the color of the dish to remain uniform without having additional black specks. Frankly, I'm not that much of a purist and appreciate the color contrast, but I wanted to give you the option.

compassionate cooks' tip

Examples of summer squash include pattypan (or "scalloped"), yellow crookneck, and zucchini.

Kale Chips

▶ *Soy-free, wheat-free*

I almost didn't include this recipe because it seems like every healthful vegan cook-book has one, but I would be negligent if I left it out. It's something I eat almost every day and is loved by all who try it, especially once you get hooked on kale.

1 bunch curly or dinosaur (Lacinato) kale

1 to 2 teaspoons olive oil, or enough to coat the kale

Pinch of salt

1 tablespoon (8 g) nutritional yeast, plus more to taste (optional)

½ teaspoon chili powder (optional)

DIRECTIONS

Preheat the toaster oven or regular oven to 350°F (180°C, or gas mark 4).

Tear or cut the kale leaves away from the thick stems and tear the leaves into bite-size pieces. Wash and thoroughly dry the leaves.

Transfer the kale to a large bowl and drizzle with the olive oil, sprinkle with the salt, and add the nutritional yeast and chili powder. With your hands or tongs, toss the leaves until fully coated.

Lay the leaves out on a baking sheet in a single layer, sprinkle them with more nutritional yeast to taste, and bake until the leaves are crisp but not burnt, 10 to 15 minutes, checking every 5 minutes or so. (See note below about removing ones that are already done.) If you're doing this in a toaster oven, you may need to work in small batches.

YIELD: 2 servings

SERVING SUGGESTION AND VARIATION

Try it with garlic salt instead of regular salt.

PER SERVING: 73 Calories; 5g Fat (56.9% calories from fat); 3g Protein; 5g Carbohydrate; 2g Dietary Fiber; 0mg Cholesterol; 87mg Sodium

compassionate cooks' tips

- I cannot emphasize how little salt and oil you need for optimum flavor. When you make these again and again, like I do, you'll find just the right ratio for you.

- I also cannot emphasize how critical the baking time is. If you bake them too little, they are just limp pieces of kale; if you bake them too long, they will burn. You may need to check halfway through the cooking time to remove the pieces that are already crispy. Continue cooking and keep a close eye on the remaining leaves.

- The other trick is not piling the kale leaves on top of one another. If you do, the leaves on the top will cook, but those on the bottom will stay moist. Make sure they're all laid out in a single layer, even if you have to cook them in more than one batch.

- Because the leaves shrink so much when cooking, you may want to double the recipe for a higher yield.

Shredded Brussels Sprouts with Apples and Pecans

▶ *Soy-free if using oil or soy-free Earth Balance, wheat-free*

Admittedly, I wasn't a fan of Brussels sprouts growing up, but as an adult, my appreciation borders on fanaticism. Here is a wonderful way to enjoy these under-eaten veggies.

2 tablespoons (30 ml) oil or nondairy butter (such as Earth Balance)

1½ pounds (685 g) Brussels sprouts, washed and shredded (cut into strips)

½ teaspoon salt, plus more to taste

1 large tart apple, cubed and unpeeled

2 medium cloves garlic, minced

1 tablespoon (20 g) maple syrup

⅓ cup (50 g) pecans, toasted and chopped

Freshly ground pepper, to taste

Juice from 1 lemon (optional)

DIRECTIONS

In a large sauté pan, heat the oil over medium heat. Add the shredded Brussels sprouts and ½ teaspoon salt and sauté for 7 to 10 minutes until the sprouts being to brighten.

Add the apple cubes, garlic, and maple syrup, and cook for 3 to 5 minutes or until the apples are heated through but not too soft.

At the end of the cooking time, add the pecans, salt and pepper to taste, and lemon juice and toss.

YIELD: 2 to 4 servings

SERVING SUGGESTIONS AND VARIATIONS

Add sautéed, baked, or caramelized tofu to make this a heartier main dish instead of a side dish.

PER SERVING: 249 Calories; 16g Fat (52.4% calories from fat); 6g Protein; 26g Carbohydrate; 8g Dietary Fiber; 0mg Cholesterol; 306mg Sodium

compassionate cooks' tip

Although it takes just a little time, it is pretty simple to shred the sprouts. Cut them in half, rest them flat side down, and cut them lengthwise into thin slices.

food lore

Brussels sprouts are neither originally from Brussels nor sprouts. They are little cabbages (in the same family as kale, collard greens, cabbage, and broccoli) most likely cultivated in ancient Rome.

did you know?

Brussels sprouts, besides boasting high amounts of vitamins C and K, contain a number of disease-fighting phytochemicals, including sulforaphane, which helps rid the body of carcinogenic substances.

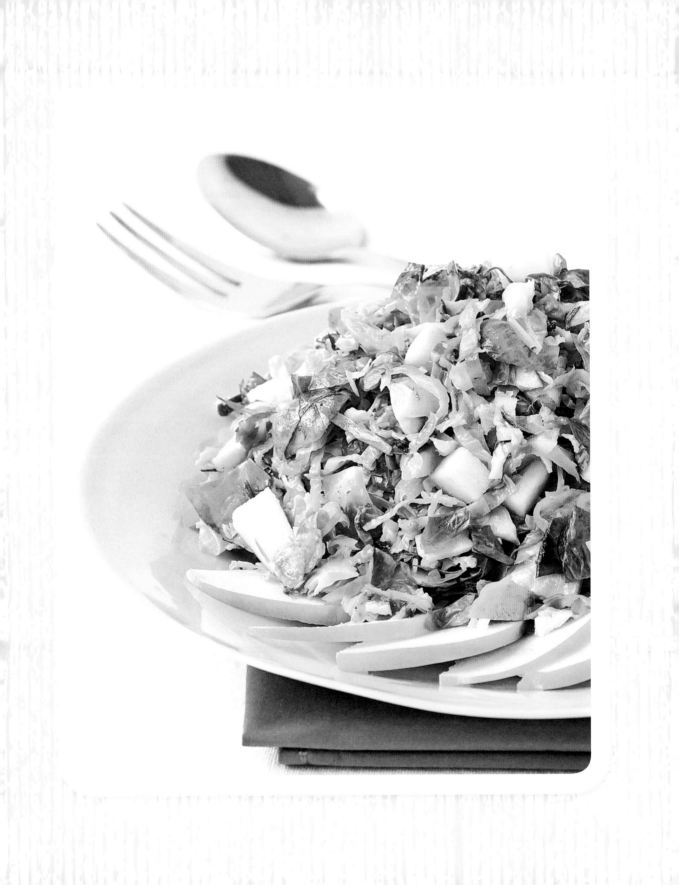

Irish Mashed Potatoes with Kale (*Colcannon*)

▶ *Wheat-free, soy-free if using soy-free Earth Balance*

A traditional Irish dish, this is a great way to add greens to your and your family's diet. After all, nobody turns down mashed potatoes! Although cabbage was originally paired with the potatoes, I can't resist an opportunity to recommend its healthier relative, kale.

2 pounds (905 g) creamy yellow potatoes, peeled and quartered

2 to 3 tablespoons (28 to 42 g) nondairy butter (such as Earth Balance), divided

Salt and freshly ground pepper, to taste

1 bunch Lacinato (aka dinosaur or cavolo nero) kale

1 tablespoon (15 ml) olive oil

1 large yellow onion, finely diced

4 cloves garlic, minced

1 tablespoon (15 ml) balsamic vinegar, preferably white

¼ cup (60 ml) nondairy milk (such as almond, soy, rice, hazelnut, hemp, or oat)

¼ teaspoon ground nutmeg

DIRECTIONS

In a large pot of water, boil the potatoes until fork-tender, about 25 minutes. Drain (reserving some of the cooking water) and transfer to a bowl for mashing. Add some of the reserved cooking water and mash by hand or with a hand mixer. Add 2 tablespoons (28 g) of the butter and salt to taste.

While the potatoes are cooking, pull the kale leaves from the thick ribs and tear into bite-size pieces. Heat the oil in a large sauté pan and add the onion. Cook over medium-low heat until golden brown, 10 to 15 minutes.

Add the kale and garlic and sauté for 10 or 12 minutes longer until the kale is tender but still chewy.

Add the vinegar and stir to combine. Season with salt and pepper to taste and remove from the heat.

In a small saucepan, bring the milk just to a boil and add the nutmeg. Stir the milk into the mashed potatoes.

Combine the mashed potatoes with the kale and onion mixture and top with the remaining 1 tablespoon (14 g) butter. Serve immediately.

YIELD: 6 servings

PER SERVING: 199 Calories; 8g Fat (33.9% calories from fat); 4g Protein; 30g Carbohydrate; 3g Dietary Fiber; 0mg Cholesterol; 7mg Sodium

compassionate cooks' tips

• Spoon the colcannon into a casserole dish and bake in a 350°F (180°C, or gas mark 4) oven for 15 minutes.

• Use leftovers to make patties, and fry in a little nondairy butter or oil. Now you've made a traditional English dish called Bubble and Squeak!

food lore

Although the word *colcannon* comes from the Irish cál *ceannann*, meaning "white-headed cabbage," any greens may be used, such as kale, leeks, or collards.

Cajun Okra

▶ *Wheat-free, soy-free*

Originally hailing from West Africa, okra most likely made its way to the United States through the human slave trade. Perfect for adding thickness to a stew (the vegetable itself is also called "gumbo"), it tends to be deep-fried in the southern United States.

1 tablespoon (15 ml) oil

1 medium yellow onion, chopped

1 bell pepper (green, red, yellow, or orange), chopped

3 cloves garlic, minced

5 large tomatoes, seeded and chopped

1 can (15 ounces, or 420 g) black-eyed peas, drained and rinsed

¼ cup (60 ml) water

2 tablespoons (8 g) chopped fresh parsley

½ teaspoon dried thyme

½ teaspoon ground cumin

¼ teaspoon chili powder

¼ teaspoon cayenne pepper

⅛ teaspoon ground cloves

Salt and freshly ground pepper, to taste

1 pound (455 g) fresh okra, stemmed and sliced into ½-inch (1.3 cm) rounds

DIRECTIONS

Heat the oil in a large soup pot. Add the onion, bell pepper, and garlic and sauté until the onion is translucent, about 7 minutes. Add the chopped tomatoes, black-eyed peas, water, parsley, thyme, cumin, chili powder, cayenne pepper, cloves, and salt and pepper to taste. Simmer for 5 minutes.

Add the okra and stir well. Simmer for 15 minutes. If the mixture gets too thick, add water as needed.

Serve over brown rice or toss with your favorite pasta.

YIELD: 2 to 4 servings

SERVING SUGGESTIONS AND VARIATIONS

Frozen okra can be used in place of fresh, and canned tomatoes can be used in place of fresh.

PER SERVING: 484 Calories; 6g Fat (10.0% calories from fat); 29g Protein; 84g Carbohydrate; 18g Dietary Fiber; 0mg Cholesterol; 45mg Sodium

food lore

Although the terms tend to be used interchangeably, there is indeed a difference between Creole and Cajun people and cuisine.

Creoles were the first European (French, Spanish, and Portuguese) settlers in New Orleans; wealthy and educated, these settlers also brought with them their chefs, influenced by and trained in European haute cuisine. Creole cuisine is thus refined and subtle, relying on rich sauces and roux.

The Cajuns, on the other hand, were French settlers who lived in an area in Nova Scotia called Acadia. ("Cajun" is a bastardization of "Acadian.") Arriving in Louisiana in about 1765 after being forced out of Acadia (now Canada) by the British, Cajuns were mostly of peasant descent with little or no education. To sustain themselves, Cajuns lived off the land and relied on local ingredients. Cajun cuisine is thus pungent and well seasoned, sometimes spicy.

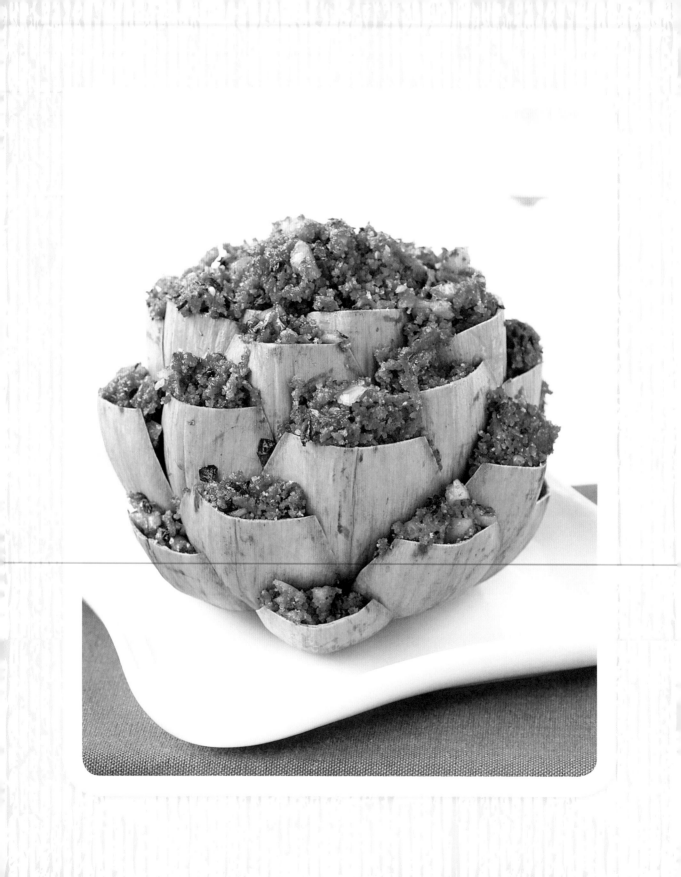

Stuffed Artichokes

▶ *Soy-free if using soy-free Earth Balance, wheat-free if using wheat-free bread crumbs*

Too many people are intimidated by this gorgeous, folate-rich vegetable (actually a flower bud). The truth is, once you learn the ins and outs (literally!) of working with an artichoke, it becomes second nature.

4 large artichokes

3 tablespoons (45 ml) oil, divided

1 yellow onion, chopped

4 cloves garlic, minced

1 cup (50 g) bread crumbs

½ cup (50 g) walnuts, toasted and finely chopped

4 medium tomatoes, seeded and diced

1 teaspoon salt

Freshly ground pepper, to taste

3 tablespoons (9 g) fresh herbs (parsley, basil, oregano, thyme), minced

1 teaspoon lemon juice

Melted nondairy butter (such as Earth Balance) or eggless aioli, for serving

DIRECTIONS

With a sharp knife, cut the stems off the artichokes so they sit flush. With scissors, cut the pointy tips off the outer artichoke leaves. In a large pot with a steamer basket, steam the whole artichokes for 25 to 45 minutes or until the leaves pull easily away and are tender at the base. The cooking time varies according to the size of your artichokes, type of steamer you use, amount of water, etc.

Meanwhile, in a large sauté pan, heat 1 tablespoon (15 ml) of the oil and sauté the onion and garlic over medium heat for about 5 minutes until the onion is soft and translucent.

Add more oil as necessary along with the bread crumbs and walnuts. Combine thoroughly with the onion and garlic mixture.

Add the tomatoes and salt, stirring them into the mixture, and season with pepper to taste. Stir in the fresh herbs and the lemon juice, adjust the seasonings, and remove from the heat. When the artichokes are done and cool enough to handle, pry open the tops with your fingers and expose the cavity into which you will spoon the mixture.

How to eat an artichoke: Pull off the outer petals and dip the bottom of each leaf—the white fleshy end—into melted nondairy butter or eggless aioli (try Wildwood's Garlic Aioli). Tightly grip the top end of the petal. Place the dipped end in your mouth, bite down, and pull the leaf through your teeth to remove the soft portion of the petal. Discard the remaining part of the petal. Continue until all the leaves are removed and the heart and choke are revealed.

How to remove the choke and eat the heart: Once you've eaten all the leaves, devoured the stuffing, and reached the choke, use a spoon to scrape the top of the heart to remove all the white feathery part (the choke). What you have left is the heart of the artichoke. Cut it into bite-size pieces and enjoy!

YIELD: 4 servings

SERVING SUGGESTIONS AND VARIATIONS

The stuffing can be made 3 days ahead, refrigerated, chilled, and covered.

PER SERVING: 319 Calories; 19g Fat (49.1% calories from fat); 10g Protein; 33g Carbohydrate; 10g Dietary Fiber; 0mg Cholesterol; 775mg Sodium

Spanish Squash Sauté *(Calabacitas)*

▶ *Oil-free if sautéing in water, soy-free, wheat-free*

A wonderful way to use the abundance of summer vegetables at your local farmers' market (or from your backyard), this is a simple dish you can prepare in advance.

1 tablespoon (15 ml) oil or water, for sautéing

1 medium yellow onion, chopped

3 cloves garlic, minced

6 cups (720 g) diced zucchini squash
   (about 3 medium squash), unpeeled

1 red, yellow, orange, or green bell pepper, diced

1 cup corn kernels (154 g fresh or 164 g frozen)

1 teaspoon chili powder

½ teaspoon ground cumin

½ teaspoon salt, or to taste

DIRECTIONS

Heat the oil in sauté pan over medium-high heat. Add the onion and garlic and cook, stirring, until translucent, about 5 minutes.

Add the zucchini and bell pepper and sauté until the vegetables are soft, about 7 minutes.

Stir in the corn, chili powder, cumin, and salt to taste until the flavors and heat are evenly distributed.

YIELD: 6 servings

SERVING SUGGESTIONS AND VARIATIONS

Serve as the filling for tostadas, tacos, or burritos; as a side dish; or as a topping for a baked potato.

PER SERVING: 73 Calories; 3g Fat (29.7% calories from fat); 3g Protein; 12g Carbohydrate; 3g Dietary Fiber; 0mg Cholesterol; 188mg Sodium

did you know?

Because color is where nutrients are saturated, you've probably surmised that the health benefits in zucchini squash reside not in the flesh but in the peel. The flesh of summer squash is white and 95 percent water, so just wash the skin and don't peel!

food lore

Calabacitas means "little squash" in Spanish.

Garlicky Greens with Pasta

▶ *Soy-free, wheat-free if using wheat-free pasta*

This is a flexible dish with many different options for greens, for pasta, for spiciness, and for the amount of garlic. It's a go-to dish for any season.

1 tablespoon (18 g) salt

2 pounds (910 g) broccoli rabe, mustard, or dandelion greens, cut into 1-inch (2.5-cm) strips

1 pound (455 g) uncooked orechiette, penne, or other favorite tube pasta

2 to 3 tablespoons (30 to 45 ml) olive oil

4 cloves garlic, minced

¼ teaspoon crushed red pepper flakes, or to taste

1 to 2 teaspoons finely chopped fresh basil leaves

2 to 4 tablespoons (18 to 35 g) toasted pine nuts

Salt and freshly ground pepper, to taste

DIRECTIONS

In a large pot, bring 2 to 3 quarts (2.2 to 3.3 L) of water to a boil. Add the salt and toss the greens into the boiling water. Cook until they are almost tender but still bright green, 8 to 10 minutes.

With a slotted spoon, remove the greens from the pot (don't discard the water) and toss them into a large bowl of ice water. After a couple of minutes in the cold water, simply drain the greens in a colander.

Return the pot of water to a boil. Add the pasta to the pot of water in which the greens were cooked. While the pasta cooks, squeeze the greens to remove as much water as possible. Toss the greens to separate them and set aside.

In a large sauté pan or wok, heat the olive oil over medium-high heat. Add the garlic and cook, stirring constantly with a wooden spoon, just until the garlic begins to turn golden brown. (Do not let it burn or the garlic will turn bitter.) Add the red pepper flakes.

Just before the pasta is done, add the drained greens to the garlic and oil and cook for 2 minutes, stirring constantly. Remove the pan from the heat.

Drain the pasta, leaving a bit of water clinging to it. Immediately add the pasta to the cooked greens still in the pan; toss well with the fresh basil and toasted pine nuts and season to taste with salt and pepper. Serve immediately.

YIELD: 4 servings

SERVING SUGGESTIONS AND VARIATIONS

The flavors are still great after storing it in the fridge overnight. If the pasta becomes dry, toss it with a little olive oil to moisten it up.

PER SERVING: 555 Calories; 15g Fat (25.2% calories from fat); 16g Protein; 87g Carbohydrate; 3g Dietary Fiber; 0mg Cholesterol; 1753mg Sodium

food lore

Garlic's reputation for warding off vampires predates Bram Stoker's 1897 classic novel, *Dracula*, which set this myth in stone (or, rather, on paper). As for the origins of this bit of folklore, it does have some truth, most likely having to do with the antibacterial property of garlic—for treating such things as *bites*.

Green Tea and Pistachio Cupcakes

▶ *Soy-free if using soy-free Earth Balance and milk*

The green color from the matcha tea is breathtaking, and these cupcakes are absolutely moist and magnificent.

CUPCAKES

2 cups (240 g) all-purpose or whole wheat pastry flour

½ to ¾ cup (100 to 150 g) granulated sugar

2 tablespoons (18 g) plus 1 teaspoon powdered green tea (such as matcha)

½ teaspoon ground cinnamon

1½ teaspoons baking powder

½ teaspoon salt

1 cup (235 ml) nondairy milk (such as almond, soy, rice, hazelnut, hemp, or oat)

⅓ cup (80 ml) canola oil

1 teaspoon pure vanilla extract

GREEN TEA FROSTING

½ cup (112 g) nonhydrogenated, nondairy butter (such as Earth Balance)

1½ cups (150 g) confectioners' sugar, sifted

1 teaspoon powdered green tea (such as matcha)

3 to 4 tablespoons (45 to 60 ml) nondairy milk (such as almond, soy, rice, hazelnut, hemp, or oat), divided

¼ teaspoon pure vanilla extract

⅛ teaspoon almond extract

½ cup (63 g) coarsely ground pistachio nuts, for topping

DIRECTIONS

To make the cupcakes, preheat the oven to 350°F (180°C, or gas mark 4). Lightly oil a muffin tin or fill with cupcake liners.

In a large bowl, thoroughly combine the flour, sugar, green tea powder, cinnamon, baking powder, and salt.

Create a well in the center of the dry ingredients. Pour in the milk, oil, and vanilla. Stir to combine, making sure you break up any large lumps and being careful not to overstir.

Distribute the batter among the 12 prepared muffin cups and bake for 20 minutes or until a toothpick inserted into the center comes out clean. Let cool on a rack.

Meanwhile, to make the frosting, with an electric hand mixer or using a fork, cream the butter until smooth. Add the sugar, green tea powder, 2 tablespoons (30 ml) of the milk, vanilla extract, and almond extract. Beat for a few minutes until the frosting is light and fluffy, adding 1 or 2 tablespoons (15 or 30 ml) more milk, if needed. Cover the icing with plastic wrap and store in the refrigerator for about 1 hour. If the icing gets too warm in the kitchen, it will be thin rather than fluffy. Store it in a covered container in the refrigerator for up to 2 weeks. Rewhip before using.

When ready to use, frost each cupcake and top with the ground pistachios.

YIELD: 12 cupcakes

PER SERVING: 295 Calories; 13g Fat (41.3% calories from fat); 2g Protein; 41g Carbohydrate; 2g Dietary Fiber; 0mg Cholesterol; 151mg Sodium

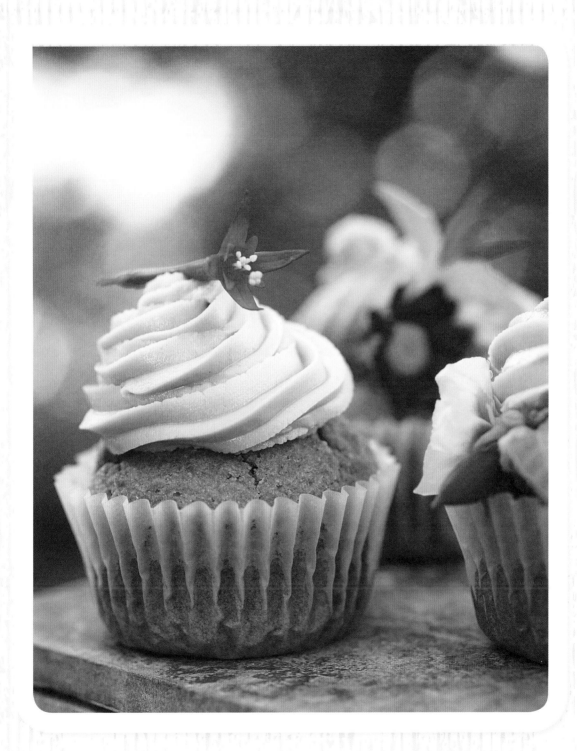

Avocado Pudding

▶ *Oil-free, soy-free, wheat-free*

The color of this creamy dessert is absolutely stunning, and although the taste and presentation are very sophisticated, it is incredibly easy to prepare. Reduce the sugar a bit, and you have a wonderful breakfast pudding that goes well with any fruit.

3 ripe avocados
⅓ cup (65 g) granulated sugar, divided
Juice of 2 lemons
Sliced kiwi or banana, for garnish

DIRECTIONS

Using a small knife, peel and core the avocados. Purée the avocado meat in a blender or food processor with 4 tablespoons (50 g) of the sugar and the lemon juice. Taste for flavor and add more sugar or lemon, if necessary, depending on your preference and the quality and ripeness of the avocados.

Serve it right away, garnished with the fruit, or chill it in the refrigerator for 30 minutes before serving.

YIELD: 4 servings

SERVING SUGGESTIONS AND VARIATIONS
• Serve in martini glasses with fruit slices as garnish on the edge of the glass.
• Serve with Caramelized Bananas (page 101).

PER SERVING: 311 Calories; 23g Fat (61.6% calories from fat); 3g Protein; 29g Carbohydrate; 4g Dietary Fiber; 0mg Cholesterol; 15mg Sodium

compassionate cooks' tips

• To speed the ripening process of avocados, place them in brown paper bags and store in a warm place until soft.

• To prevent avocados from turning brown once you've cut them in half, spread a few drops of lemon juice on plastic wrap, and seal the avocado tightly, smoothing away any air bubbles. If it still browns slightly, it is most likely only a very thin layer on the top and can be cut away before using.

did you know?

Disease-fighting compounds such as lutein, beta-carotene, and vitamin E are abundant in avocados, and fiber is not far behind (with one half providing 10 percent of the Daily Value).

food lore

I often say that it's not meat we crave—it's fat and salt (and texture, flavor, and familiarity). Avocados prove my point. Because of their rich, creamy texture, avocados used to be known as "poor man's butter." Not everyone could afford to keep "livestock," but a few avocado trees in the backyard were all they needed. Even today some people use these so-called "butter pears" in lieu of dairy-based butter, though the reason is to increase nutrients rather than save money.

Green Smoothies

▸ *Wheat-free, oil-free, soy-free*

Admittedly, it's very difficult to create a "recipe" for smoothies, because there are so many options and variations. Apples provide soluble and insoluble fiber as well as antioxidants and nutritional goodness, bananas add much-needed potassium as well as thickness, flaxseed adds the ever-important omega-3 fatty acids, and greens—well, you just can't say enough good things about greens.

1 ripe banana, preferably frozen chunks from the freezer

1 or 2 apples, quartered (not peeled)

1 cup (15 g) pineapple chunks (frozen adds creaminess)

2 loose cups (60 g) spinach (or kale or chard or other greens)

½-inch (2.5 cm) piece ginger, peeled

1 tablespoon (7 g) ground flaxseed

2 dates, pitted

1½ cups (353 ml) cold water

¼ cup (60 ml) apple, pineapple, or orange juice

DIRECTIONS

Blend all the ingredients until fully combined. Make it thinner or thicker with more or less juice, depending on your preference.

YIELD: 2 servings

PER SERVING: 206 Calories; 2g Fat (8.6% calories from fat); 3g Protein; 49g Carbohydrate; 7g Dietary Fiber; 0mg Cholesterol; 31mg Sodium

compassionate cooks' tips

- Frozen bananas are perfect for smoothies, because they add cold and creaminess. Peel ripe bananas, break them into chunks, and store them in the freezer in a plastic bag or plastic container. You can also freeze them whole and in their peel. (You'll have to wait for them to thaw before being able to break them up. They'll turn black on the outside when they're frozen, but they're still good.)

- If you add blueberries, your green smoothie will turn an unattractive gray.

- Any blender works well, though you may need to scrape down the sides periodically. Please see Resources and Recommendations for my favorite kitchen items.

Kiwi Banana Muffins

▶ *Soy-free if using soy-free Earth Balance, oil-free*

Between the bananas and the kiwifruit, these little muffins pack a super potassium punch.

2 cups (240 g) all-purpose flour
1 teaspoon baking powder
¼ teaspoon baking soda
½ teaspoon salt
Zest from 1 medium orange
3 ripe bananas, peeled
8 ripe kiwis, peeled, divided
½ cup (112 g) nondairy butter (such as Earth Balance), softened
⅓ cup (66 g) granulated sugar

DIRECTIONS

Preheat the oven to 350°F (180°C, or gas mark 4). Lightly oil a muffin tin or fill with cupcake liners.

In a large bowl, stir together the flour, baking powder, baking soda, salt, and orange zest. Set aside.

In a medium bowl or in a food processor or blender, mash (or purée) the bananas and 5 of the kiwis until smooth. Add the butter and sugar and stir to combine.

Chop the remaining 3 kiwis into bite-size pieces.

Fold the wet ingredients into the dry ingredients, add the chopped kiwi, and stir to combine.

Spoon the batter into the individual muffin tins and bake for 15 to 20 minutes or until a toothpick inserted into the center of the muffins comes out clean. This might take longer if your muffins are on the larger side.

Cool for 10 minutes on wire rack.

YIELD: 12 muffins

PER SERVING: 216 Calories; 7g Fat (30.6% calories from fat); 3g Protein; 35g Carbohydrate; 3g Dietary Fiber; 0mg Cholesterol; 238mg Sodium

food lore

Native to China, the kiwifruit was originally known as the Chinese gooseberry. New Zealand exporters changed the name in the middle of the twentieth century, naming it for that country's national bird and the colloquial name for the New Zealand people.

compassionate cooks' tips

- The 5 kiwis you use for the purée should yield about ½ cup (125 g). Use more kiwis if yours are small and not providing that much purée.

- I like the kiwi somewhat textured and not mushy, which is why I suggest some puréed and some chopped.

did you know?

In addition to their high content of vitamin C and potassium, kiwis are one of the richest sources of lutein and zeaxanthin.

WAYS TO INCREASE GREEN FOODS

- Make a Green Smoothie (page 129).

- Drink green tea (see "The Many Colors of Tea," pages 216 and 217).

- Add frozen or fresh sweet peas to cooked rice.

- Use large collard leaves as a roll-up (instead of a tortilla). Spread some pesto on the leaf and add thin strips of cucumber, carrot, and other favorite vegetables. Roll it up and eat!

- Eat at least one large salad at one meal every day. Vary the greens to include lettuce, spinach, or a mixture of greens. Have fun and add as many green veggies you can come up with: green bell pepper, snow or snap peas, green tomatoes, fennel, shredded Brussels sprouts, green cabbage, avocado, and basil.

- Steam greens, such as kale, chard, collard greens, or spinach and serve as an extra side dish with your evening meal.

- Add fresh herbs to all of your recipes for extra flavor and nutrition.

- Keep broccoli chopped up into florets to easily grab from the fridge and eat as a snack. Dip it into healthful hummus.

- Snack on my favorite olive of all time: the gorgeous blue/green meaty Castelvetrano olive. Find them fresh in large natural grocery stores or jarred in Italian grocers.

- Snack on edamame beans. Buy them frozen, and cook in boiling water for 5 minutes.

- Make my famous Garlic and Greens Soup demonstrated by me in a video at www.compassionatecooks.com.

- Crispy kale makes a great snack. See the recipe for Kale Chips on page 117.

- Mash steamed broccoli into mashed potatoes.

- Add julienned kale, chard, or any leafy green to marinara sauce before serving over pasta.

- If you're going to eat pasta or flour tortillas anyway, why not choose the spinach-infused green versions?

- Eat celery with peanut butter as a snack.

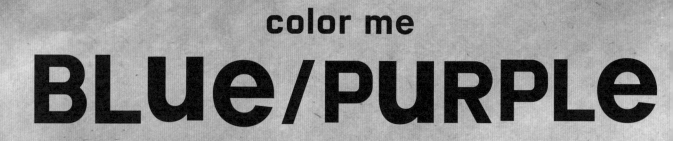

color me
BLUE/PURPLE

FLOWER-INSPIRED POWER

Did you know that analysis of the latest data from the National Health and Nutrition Examination Study, a survey of eating and health habits, found that adults who eat purple and blue fruits and vegetables have a *reduced risk* for both high blood pressure and *low* HDL cholesterol (the "good" kind) and that they are also less likely to be overweight? Did you also know that purple and blue foods make up only 3 percent of the average American's fruit and vegetable intake?

Let's back up. Why would the colors blue and purple have such a positive effect on human health? Well, think about the plants themselves and the hours and hours of direct sunlight they are subjected to day in and day out. Now, that's a good thing (after all, photosynthesis gives them life), but it can also damage them by generating free radicals (those nasty, unstable molecules).

Free radicals can be just as damaging to plants as they are to humans, and antioxidants are the protectors of both. Antioxidants show up as the protective pigments in the plant—the sunblock, if you will—and they vary according to the plant and its colors.

The most prominent antioxidants in blue and purple plants are a class of pigments called *anthocyanins*. This is where our best friend etymology (the study of the origins of words) comes in. The word *anthocyanin* comes from the Greek words *anthos*, meaning "flower," and *kyanos*, meaning "dark blue." These pigments span the red-blue-purple spectrum, ranging from burgundy and fuchsia to periwinkle and sapphire.

What makes these pigments even more endearing is the floral names they were given in honor of their associations with flowers (providing the red in roses and the blue in violets). Specific types of anthocyanins include *delphinidin* (named for delphiniums), *petunidin* (for petunias), *peonidin* (for peonies), *rosinidin* (for roses), *chrysanthenin* (for chrysanthemums), *tulipinin* (for tulips), and so on.

Now, anthocyanins aren't the only antioxidants providing protection in our blue and purple foods, but they're the most easily identifiable ones. In the following recipes, you'll also be drowning in the *saponins* in your eggplant, *resveratrol* in your purple grapes, *ellagic acid* in your blueberries and blackberries, vitamin C in your purple plums, *perillyl alcohol* in your culinary lavender, *phenolic acids* in your figs, and *quercetin* in your raisins, all of which provide protection against disease.

Also in this section are foods that may be familiar in another color family but that have a blue side as well. After all, purple pole beans are flashier than their green counterparts, purple cauliflower is more exciting than white, purple potatoes will give you a new respect for tired tubers, and purple kale will have you reaching for more. However, the more familiar versions of these veggies can easily be used in place of the violet variations.

Have fun, change things up, and eat until you're blue in the face—well, sorta. Enjoy!

Radicchio Fennel Salad with Caper Dressing

▶ *Soy-free, wheat-free*

Enjoy the range of textures and tastes in this beautiful and flavorful salad.

1 head radicchio, shredded

½ head green leaf lettuce or romaine, shredded

2 fennel bulbs, cut into 1-inch (2.5 cm) strips

¼ cup (60 ml) olive oil

Juice from 1 lemon

10 Italian- or Greek-style black olives, pitted and sliced, divided

1 tablespoon (9 g) capers, rinsed

¼ teaspoon salt

Dash of freshly ground black pepper

1 teaspoon granulated sugar or agave nectar

2 tablespoons (5 g) finely chopped fresh basil

Fennel tops, for garnish

DIRECTIONS

Add the radicchio, lettuce, and fennel to a large salad bowl. Set aside.

Combine the olive oil, lemon juice, 5 of the olives, and the capers in a blender. Process until smooth. Taste and add salt, pepper, and sugar, as necessary.

Just before serving, toss the dressing with the salad ingredients, adding the remaining 5 olives and the basil. You may also add more capers in addition to the ones you used for the dressing.

Serve right away, garnished with the fennel tops.

YIELD: 4 servings

SERVING SUGGESTIONS AND VARIATIONS

To add a little more blue/purple to this dish, switch out the green basil for purple basil.

PER SERVING: 179 Calories; 16g Fat (77.6% calories from fat); 1g Protein; 9g Carbohydrate; 3g Dietary Fiber; 0mg Cholesterol; 489mg Sodium

compassionate cooks' tip

Radicchio tends to oxidize (turn brown) rather quickly, so don't chop it too far in advance before serving.

did you know?

Somewhat bitter-tasting, radicchio is a purplish-red leafy vegetable related to chicory that adds color and crunch to any mixed salad. It's very popular in Italy and can be eaten raw or grilled and roasted.

advance preparation required

Purple Cabbage Salad

▶ *Soy-free, wheat-free*

The purple cabbage becomes even brighter when it marinates for a bit (turning the marinade a gorgeous deep purple). Keep it crisp by preparing it no more than a few hours ahead of serving.

1 head purple cabbage, shredded
1 small red onion, sliced
3 scallions, chopped
1 jalapeño pepper, minced
½ cup (75 g) raisins
¼ cup (60 ml) orange juice
¼ cup (60 ml) apple cider vinegar
1 tablespoon (15 ml) olive oil
2 tablespoons (30 ml) agave nectar
1 orange, peeled and sliced into ½-inch
   (1.3-cm) segments
1 pineapple, cut into chunks
¼ teaspoon salt
Dash of chili powder
¼ to ½ cup (40 to 75 g) toasted hazelnuts,
   coarsely chopped
¼ cup (35 g) toasted sunflower seeds

DIRECTIONS

In a large bowl, toss together the cabbage, red onion, scallions, jalapeño pepper, and raisins. Add the orange juice, apple cider vinegar, olive oil, agave nectar, orange segments, pineapple chunks, salt, and chili powder. Toss until well combined and refrigerate for at least 1 hour.

Just before serving, add the hazelnuts and sunflower seeds and stir to combine. I prefer adding the nuts and seeds at this point to retain their crunch.

YIELD: 6 to 8 servings

SERVING SUGGESTIONS AND VARIATIONS

• For extra color and crunch, add grated carrots and sliced radishes.
• If fresh pineapple is not available, canned pineapple can be used. (Look for pineapple in its own juice, not with added sweeteners.)
• So that they don't get stained blue and stay a vibrant yellow, add the pineapple at the end of tossing all the ingredients together.

PER SERVING: 166 Calories; 5g Fat (25.9% calories from fat); 3g Protein; 31g Carbohydrate; 5g Dietary Fiber; 0mg Cholesterol; 91mg Sodium

did you know?

The anthocyanins (the phytochemicals that produce the blue color in cabbage and other plants) change their hue depending on the pH level (acidity or alkalinity) of their environment. For instance, the anthocyanin turns bright pink in acids, reddish-purple in neutral solutions, and green in alkaline or basic solutions. The acidic vinegar and orange juice in this recipe help the cabbage retain its bright color.

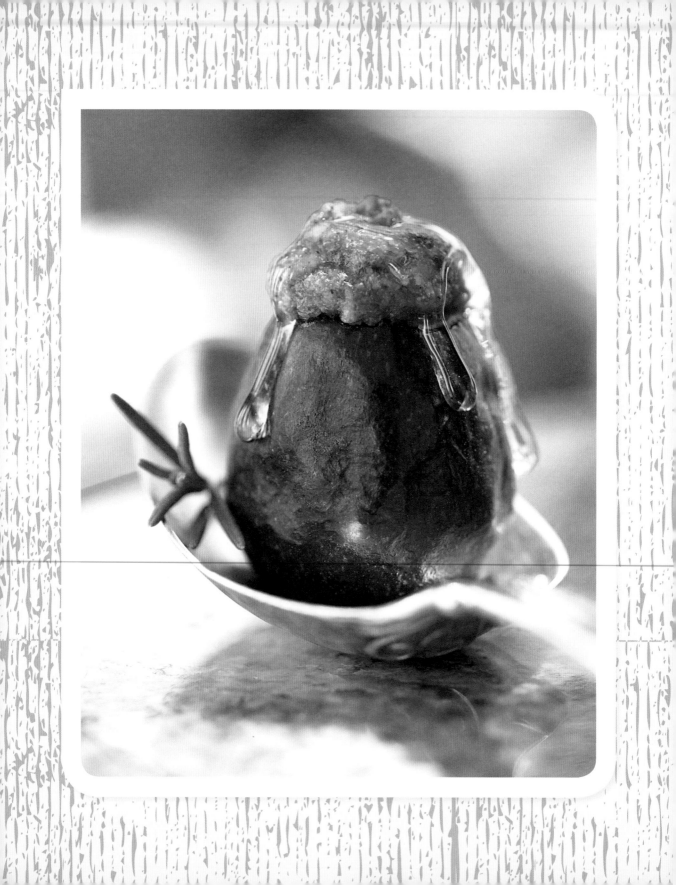

advance preparation required

Figs Stuffed with Rosemary and Walnut-Cashew Cream

▶ *Wheat-free*

This simple yet delicious cashew cream comes from my friends Barry and Jennifer Jones-Horton of Local Love, an organic vegan food services company in Oakland, CA.

1 cup (145 g) raw cashews

1 tablespoon (15 ml) olive oil, plus additional oil for brushing

½ yellow onion, finely chopped

1 teaspoon yellow/light miso

1 tablespoon (15 ml) lemon juice

1 tablespoon (15 ml) water

¼ cup (25 g) raw walnuts

1 tablespoon (12 g) nutritional yeast

1 tablespoon (2 g) rosemary, minced

Salt and freshly ground pepper, to taste

12 Black Mission figs or other figs of your choice, stemmed

Agave nectar, for drizzling

Rosemary sprigs, for garnish

DIRECTIONS

Soak the cashews overnight in just enough water to completely cover them. The next day, drain and rinse the cashews. Set aside.

In a medium sauté pan, heat the olive oil and sauté the onion until translucent and tender, 5 to 7 minutes. Place the soaked cashews, sautéed onion, miso, lemon juice, and water in a blender and process until smooth. Transfer to a bowl.

In a food processor, pulse the walnuts until coarsely chopped. Stir the chopped walnuts, nutritional yeast, and minced rosemary into the cashew mixture. Taste and season with salt and pepper. At this point, you may store the cream in the refrigerator for up to 3 days or continue on to stuff and roast the figs.

When ready to prepare and serve the stuffed figs, preheat the oven to 425°F (220°C, or gas mark 7). Lightly oil a glass roasting pan.

Set each fig upright on the cutting board and working from the top down, carefully cut crosswise into the top of each fig, as if you were quartering it, but making sure not to cut all the way through. You don't want to cut them all the way to separate them; you want them to remain intact but open enough to pipe in the creamy filling.

You may either spoon 1 tablespoon (15 g) of the cashew cream into each cavity or transfer the cashew cream to a piping bag and pipe 1 tablespoon (15 g) of the cream into the cavity of each fig.

Transfer the filled figs to the prepared roasting pan, brush or lightly spray the figs with a little oil, and roast for about 12 minutes or until the figs are soft.

Drizzle on some agave nectar just before serving and garnish the serving platter with rosemary sprigs.

YIELD: 12 servings

PER SERVING: 109 Calories; 6g Fat (46.4% calories from fat); 2g Protein; 13g Carbohydrate; 3g Dietary Fiber; 0mg Cholesterol; 63mg Sodium

Grilled Purple Pole Beans

▶ *Wheat-free, soy-free*

Certainly green or even yellow pole beans work just as well, but purple beans add anthocyanin-rich charm! Create a visual work of art by using all three colors.

1 pound (455 g) purple or green pole beans
1 to 2 tablespoons (15 to 30 ml) olive oil
2 or 3 cloves garlic, minced
Salt and freshly ground pepper, to taste
Juice from ½ lemon

DIRECTIONS

Snap off the tips and stems of each bean, wash under running water, and pat dry.

Light the grill to a medium flame and adjust the grill pan or foil.

Transfer the beans to a large bowl and toss them with the olive oil, garlic, salt, and pepper. Make sure they're evenly coated before transferring them to the grill.

Grill for 10 to 15 minutes, until the beans are crisp-tender with spots of golden brown. Be sure to lay the beans crosswise across the grill's grate to prevent them from falling through.

Stir the beans every few minutes to make sure they cook evenly and don't burn.

Remove from the grill and squeeze some lemon juice over them. Toss and serve.

YIELD: 4 servings

PER SERVING: 107 Calories; 7g Fat (62.0% calories from fat); trace Protein; 9g Carbohydrate; 2g Dietary Fiber; 0mg Cholesterol; 408mg Sodium

did you know?

Some popular pole beans are Kentucky Blue, Kentucky Wonder, and Blue Lake. One purple variety is called Purple Podded. Yellow or "wax" beans, such as the Beurre de Rocquencourt, are also available and can be used for this recipe as well. Generally, purple, yellow, and green beans are identical in taste and texture.

compassionate cooks' tip

Purple beans tend to become green once they're cooked. One way to bring out their color is to add lemon juice to them while they're cooking. You can also try blanching them in water that has a pinch of baking soda in it.

food lore

Pole beans are beans that are bred to grow as vines to climb poles or trellises. One of the staples in my garden, they are easy to grow, because the beans tend to be quite prolific, even on the smallest plant.

Purple Cauliflower Soup

▶ *Soy-free, wheat-free*

This is a very beautiful soup no matter what color cauliflower you use, but try and find purple or orange for a special presentation. The flavor is virtually the same, though you will be consuming different antioxidants, depending on the color you use.

1 tablespoon (15 ml) water, for sautéing

1 large yellow onion, diced

2 cloves garlic, minced

1 large head purple, orange, or white cauliflower, cut into medium chunks

1 large or 2 medium yellow potatoes, peeled and diced

5½ cups (1295 ml) vegetable stock

½ teaspoon truffle or chile oil

Salt and freshly ground pepper, to taste

Chopped scallions or parsley, for garnish

DIRECTIONS

Heat the water in a sauté pan and sauté the onion until translucent, about 5 minutes. Add the garlic and cook for 1 to 2 minutes longer.

Add the cauliflower, potatoes, and vegetable stock.

Cook the soup over medium heat until the potatoes are fork-tender, about 25 minutes. Add the truffle oil and stir to combine.

Transfer to a blender and blend until smooth or use an immersion blender directly in the pot. Add salt and pepper to taste and serve hot, garnished with the green scallions for a contrasting color.

YIELD: 4 servings, or 8 cups

SERVING SUGGESTIONS AND VARIATIONS

Instead of adding the oil to the soup before blending, drizzle it on the finished soup just before serving for a pretty presentation.

PER SERVING: 103 Calories; 2g Fat (14.0% calories from fat); 2g Protein; 21g Carbohydrate; 2g Dietary Fiber; 0mg Cholesterol; 1377mg Sodium

compassionate cooks' tip

I happen to like puréeing my soups in my high-speed blender because I love them nice and creamy. I also appreciate the convenience of immersion blenders; however, my only qualm about them is that if you've added too much water or stock than needed to create the right consistency, you can't rectify this once you've blended it. You have less control over the thickness/thinness of the soup. At least when you use a blender, you can add to it as much or as little water or stock as necessary to create the perfect consistency.

advance preparation required

Chilled Blueberry Mango Soup

▶ *Soy-free if using soy-free yogurt, wheat-free, oil-free*

Enjoy this totally fat-free but filling soup that makes a striking appearance at a summer dinner with friends. Decadent though they are (fried in oil), the Blueberry Croutons (page 149) definitely put this soup over the top, providing flavor, texture, and additional nutritional benefits.

½ cup (120 ml) fresh orange juice
  (1 large orange)
¾ cup (175 ml) pineapple juice or white
  grape juice
¼ cup (50 g) granulated sugar
2 cups (290 g) fresh blueberries (or frozen,
  thawed, with their juice [310 g])
¼ cup mango chunks (frozen, thawed,
  or fresh)
1 container (6 ounces, or 175 g) plain or
  vanilla nondairy yogurt
1 recipe Blueberry Croutons (page 149),
  for garnish

DIRECTIONS

In a saucepan, bring the orange juice, pineapple juice, and sugar to a boil. Allow to boil for about 1 minute, stirring constantly. Add the blueberries and mango chunks and cook for 1 minute longer. Remove from the heat and let cool.

Add the blueberry mixture along with the yogurt to a blender pitcher. Purée until smooth and chill for at least 2 hours or overnight. (It will thicken as it cools.) Pour into bowls and garnish with the Blueberry Croutons.

YIELD: 4 servings

SERVING SUGGESTIONS AND VARIATIONS

• Wonderfully light and easy to prepare, fruit soups are incredibly versatile. Not only do they make a great first course (particularly nice at a brunch or summer lunch), but they can also be served as a dessert, snack, a light meal on a hot summer night, or as a smoothie for breakfast.
• Garnish the soup with some finely chopped mango or spear a couple of mango wedges on the side of the bowl. Add a sprig of mint for another color contrast.

PER SERVING: 427 Calories; 12g Fat (25.1% calories from fat); 6g Protein; 77g Carbohydrate; 5g Dietary Fiber; 0mg Cholesterol; 240mg Sodium.

compassinnate cooks' tip

Reduce the amount of sugar if it's too sweet or if using sweetened yogurt.

food lore

Chilled fruit soups are a summer tradition in Scandinavian and Eastern European cuisines. Seasonal berries and stone fruits, such as cherries and apricots, are the most common, though dried fruits are also sometimes used.

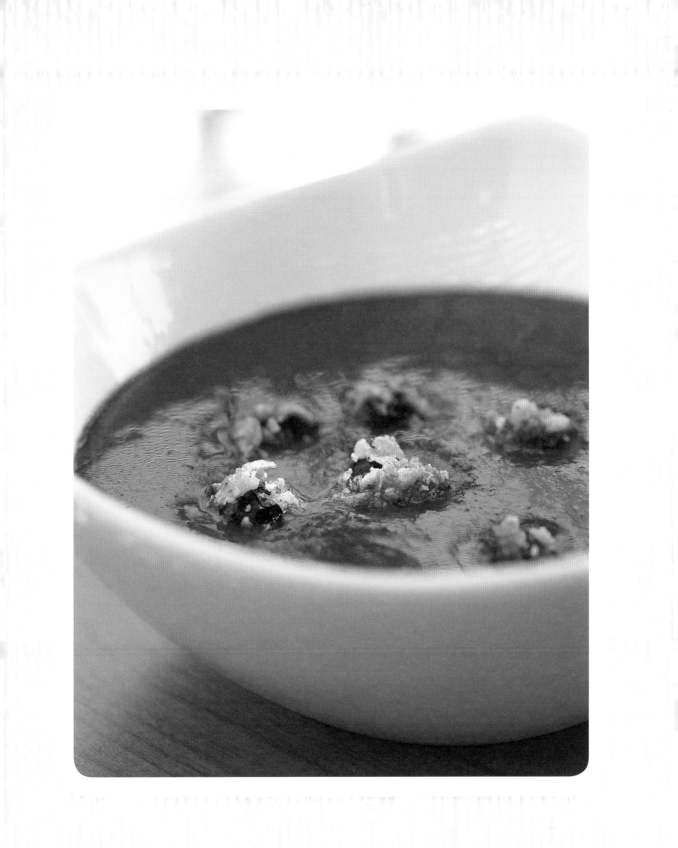

BLUEBERRIES: A SUPER SUPERFOOD

One of the few fruits native to North America, blueberries were revered by American Indians of the Northeast, who gathered them from the forests and bogs, enjoying them fresh and also preserving them for sustenance in the winter months.

Calling them "star berries" because of the perfect five-pointed star apparent on the blossom end of each berry, Native Americans also used the blueberry—and other parts of the plant—for medicinal purposes. They made tea from the leaves to help the blood, juice from the berries to treat coughs, and medicine from the roots and leaves for other ailments and to aid women during childbirth. The juice was also used as dye for baskets and food, and dried blueberries were added to stews and soups to add flavor and texture.

Scientists are beginning to demonstrate in the lab what the Native Americans already knew in nature: that the blueberry is indeed a special berry with very healthful properties. Although I'm generally reluctant to use hyperbole when it comes to making nutrition claims about a particular food, it is indeed appropriate to call blueberries a "superfood" without exaggeration.

The blueberry is a "superfood" not only because of its high vitamin C content (1 cup [145 g] yields 32 percent of the Daily Value of vitamin C) but also because of the number of antioxidants it contains, which come from two main sources: chlorogenic acid and anthocyanins.

In some fruits, it is typical to find three, four, or perhaps five different anthocyanins, but blueberries can have as many as twenty-five or thirty. It's this *concentration* that that puts one plant food over another in terms of health benefits, and this is the case with blueberries. The anthocyanins are not different or stronger or better in blueberries than in any other food; there are just so many of them in such large concentrations in these little gems.

And where is this concentration? In the flesh? No. It's the skin! If you open up a blueberry, you'll notice that they're actually *green* inside, not blue. (European *bilberries* have pigments in their flesh as well as their skin, so they may be even healthier.)

So, add blueberries to your diet each and every day (in smoothies, as a snack, in salads, in oatmeal) and experience this superfood.

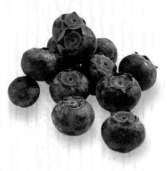

Purple Kale and White Bean Soup

▶ *Oil-free if using water to sauté, soy-free, wheat-free*

Of course, you can use green kale (dinosaur, Lacinato, or curly) for this soup, but the purple imparts a beautiful color and forces you to choose a type of kale you might not otherwise have tried.

2 tablespoons (30 ml) water or oil, for sautéing

2 medium yellow onions, diced

3 ribs celery, finely chopped

2 carrots, finely chopped

¼ teaspoon crushed red pepper flakes

1 sprig fresh rosemary

¼ teaspoon salt, plus extra, to taste

1 tablespoon (16 g) tomato paste

1 bunch purple kale, stems and ribs discarded, leaves chopped into 1-inch (2.5 cm) pieces

8 cups (1880 ml) vegetable stock

1 can (15 ounces, or 420 g) white beans (navy, cannellini), drained and rinsed

Freshly ground pepper, to taste

DIRECTIONS

Heat the water in a large soup pot over medium-low heat. Add the onions and cook, stirring occasionally, until soft and translucent, about 7 minutes. Add the celery, carrots, red pepper flakes, and rosemary sprig. Season with the ¼ teaspoon salt.

Cook, stirring occasionally, until the vegetables soften and become fragrant, about 5 minutes. Add the tomato paste and combine thoroughly with the vegetables, cooking for about 2 minutes.

Add the kale, vegetable stock, and beans. Bring to a boil over medium-high heat. Reduce the heat to a simmer and cook until the kale is tender, 15 to 20 minutes.

Remove the rosemary sprig, add pepper and salt to taste, and serve.

YIELD: 4 to 6 servings

PER SERVING: 184 Calories; 6g Fat (29.7% calories from fat); 6g Protein; 27g Carbohydrate; 5g Dietary Fiber; 0mg Cholesterol; 1413mg Sodium

food lore

Long known as the herb of remembrance and memory, rosemary was worn by students in ancient Greece while they studied for exams. Modern research indicates there may be something to this. Carnosic acid, an antioxidant in rosemary, fights off free radical damage in the brain, protecting it from stroke and neuro-degenerative conditions such as Alzheimer's disease.

did you know?

The name rosemary derives from the Latin word *rosmarinus*, which means "dew" (*ros*) and "sea" (*marinus*), or "dew of the sea," for its propensity to grow near the sea.

Purple Potato Soup

▶ *Soy-free if using soy-free milk, wheat-free, and oil-free if sautéing in water*

Although the flavor is what you would expect from a creamy potato soup, this one is all about the color. If you can't find purple potatoes, any potato would work well, but the purple just makes it extraordinary.

1 tablespoon (15 ml) oil or water, for sautéing

1 yellow onion, chopped

2 cloves garlic, minced

2 pounds (905 g) purple potatoes, peeled and quartered

1 small head cauliflower, cut into florets

2 cups (470 ml) vegetable stock (low-sodium if using canned)

1½ cups (355 ml) nondairy milk (such as almond, soy, rice, hazelnut, hemp, or oat)

Salt and freshly ground pepper, to taste

Chives, for garnish

DIRECTIONS

Heat the oil in a soup pot over medium heat and saute the onion until translucent, about 5 minutes. Add the garlic and cook for a few minutes longer until the garlic turns golden brown.

Add the potatoes, cauliflower, and vegetable stock. Cover, bring to a boil, and then reduce to a simmer and cook until the potatoes are cooked through, about 20 minutes.

Once the potatoes are fork-tender, stir in the milk and cook until heated through, about 10 minutes longer.

Purée the soup using an immersion blender, or transfer to a blender and blend until smooth. Taste, and add salt and pepper as needed.

Serve in individual bowls, preferably white, to bring out the color of the soup. Snip some chives on top of each serving as a garnish.

YIELD: 4 servings, or 8 cups (1880 ml)

PER SERVING: 276 Calories; 6g Fat (20.5% calories from fat); 3g Protein; 47g Carbohydrate; 5g Dietary Fiber; 0mg Cholesterol; 530mg Sodium

compassionate cooks' tips

- 6 or 7 medium potatoes equal roughly 2 pounds (905 g).

- There's a good chance you'll find purple potatoes at your local farmers' market, especially in the fall and winter. Otherwise, try a specialty market that carries more "exotic" produce.

- Some purple potatoes are purple only on the outside—on the skin. Others are purple all the way through to the flesh. For a purple-colored soup, choose the latter.

advance preparation required

Blueberry Ketchup

▶ *Soy-free, wheat-free, oil-free*

Having undergone centuries of variations, ketchup as we know it today is characterized by its sweet vinegary taste rather than by the salty recipe it's originally based on. This healthier version boasts the powerful phytochemicals found in blueberries.

2½ cups (375 g) fresh or frozen
  blueberries, thawed
2 tablespoons (20 g) minced shallot
1¼ cups (250 g) granulated sugar
½ cup (120 ml) red wine vinegar
2 tablespoons (12 g) minced fresh ginger
1 tablespoon (15 ml) lime juice
¼ teaspoon salt
¼ teaspoon freshly ground pepper

DIRECTIONS

Place the blueberries, shallot, sugar, vinegar, ginger, lime juice, salt, and pepper in a large saucepan over medium-high heat. Stir until the sugar dissolves, about 5 minutes.

Reduce the heat to medium-low and simmer, stirring occasionally, until the blueberries have mostly broken down and the sauce has thickened somewhat, 20 to 30 minutes. Spoon into glass jars or a large bowl and refrigerate until chilled and thickened even more, about 4 hours. It will keep in the refrigerator for up to 2 weeks or in the freezer for up to 1 month.

YIELD: 20 servings, about 2 tablespoons (30 g) each

SERVING SUGGESTIONS AND VARIATIONS

- The ketchup might be rather thick; if so, bring it to room temperature and stir.
- Use as jam and spread on toast or biscuits.
- Maximize your color consumption by serving it with Carrot Fries (page 59) and Beet Burgers (page 34).

PER SERVING: 58 Calories; trace Fat (1.1% calories from fat); trace Protein; 15g Carbohydrate; 1g Dietary Fiber; 0mg Cholesterol; 27mg Sodium

food lore

The tomato-based ketchup with which we are familiar today is different from the Chinese condiment (*ke-tsiap*) on which it was based. "Ketchup" originated in China, made its way to Malaysia (*kechap*), then Indonesia (*ketjap*), then Europe by way of Dutch and British seamen in the 1600s. Originally more akin to soy sauce or Worcestershire sauce, its saltiness was its defining characteristic. Brits created their own varieties, including their favorite made with mushrooms, and tomatoes were finally added in the 1700s. By the 1800s, ketchup was also known as tomato soy.

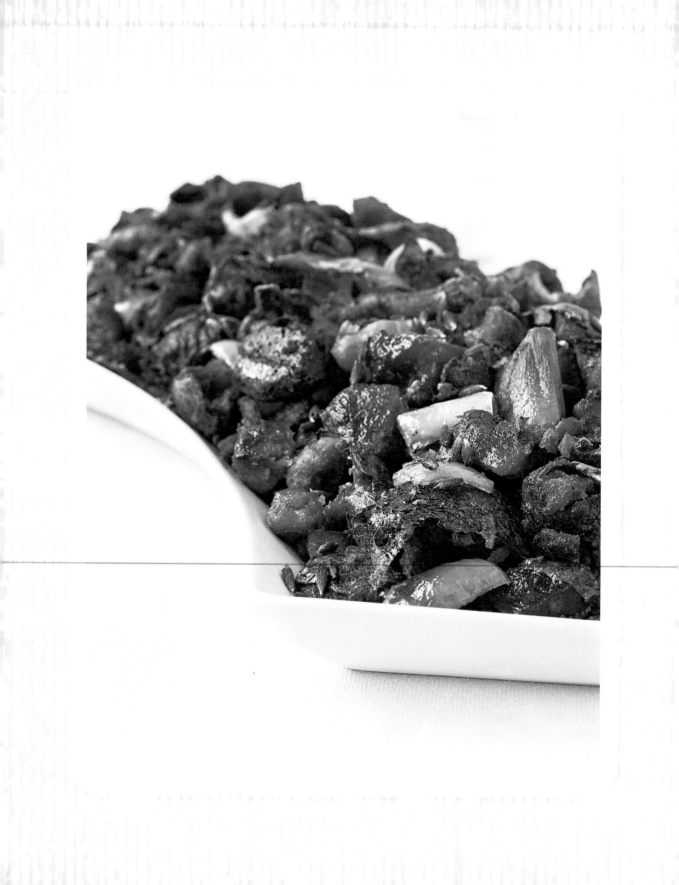

Lavender-Roasted Purple Potatoes and Purple Onions

▶ *Soy-free, wheat-free*

Lavender imparts a lovely flavor evocative of spring but can taste like perfume if overused. I find the amount used here to be perfect, resulting in a distinct but subtle taste of this hot-weather plant.

1½ pounds (685 g) purple potatoes
¼ cup (60 ml) olive oil
6 cloves garlic, minced or pressed
2 tablespoons (10 g) dried culinary lavender
2 teaspoons (3 g) fresh thyme
3 large red/purple onions, peeled, halved, and quartered
Salt and freshly ground pepper, to taste
1 tablespoon (5 g) pink peppercorns (optional)
Juice from 1 lemon or lime

DIRECTIONS

Preheat the oven to 400°F (200°C, or gas mark 6).

Boil or steam the potatoes until they are just fork-tender. If the potatoes are on the small side, you may boil them while they're still whole and unpeeled; if they're larger, quarter them first.

Meanwhile, combine the olive oil, garlic, lavender, and thyme in a bowl. Set aside.

When the potatoes are done and still warm, transfer them to a cutting board and give each one a smash with a potato masher or mallet. Add them to a large bowl, along with the onions, separating the onions into strips with your hands.

Pour the olive oil mixture over the onions and potatoes and toss to thoroughly coat (I prefer to use my hands to ensure even coverage). Season with salt and pepper.

Transfer the mixture to a baking sheet, sprinkle on the pink peppercorns (see note below), and place in the preheated oven for 25 to 35 minutes, turning the pan halfway through cooking. They're done when the potatoes and onions are golden brown and crispy.

Remove from the oven and immediately squeeze the lemon juice over the potatoes and onions. The potatoes will brighten up upon contact with the citrus juice. Serve warm or at room temperature.

YIELD: 4 servings

SERVING SUGGESTIONS AND VARIATIONS

- Add other vegetables or replace some of the onions with baby potatoes, carrots, or fennel.
- Use yellow potatoes and onions instead of purple.
- I found pink peppercorns in my local specialty foods store. They contrast beautifully with the purple potatoes and make for a special presentation.

PER SERVING: 305 Calories; 14g Fat (43.0% calories from fat); 1g Protein; 40g Carbohydrate; 4g Dietary Fiber; 0mg Cholesterol; 13mg Sodium

compassionate cooks' tip

The most familiar of this gorgeous-colored tuber is the Peruvian purple potato, which originated in Peru, the birthplace of all potatoes. Peru began cultivating potatoes between 3,000 and 2,000 BCE, from which they spread to Spain and then all over Europe. Today, China is the top potato producer, with Russia, India, and the United States following.

POTATO VARIETIES

by use
Best for Baking: Russet, Goldrush, Norkotah, Long White, White Rose, California Long White, Idaho

Best for Boiling: Round white, round red, yellow, red, salad potato, La Soda, Red La Rouge, Red Pontiac, Red Norland, Red Bliss, Yellow Finn, Ruby Crescent, Australian Crescent

Best for Roasting: Fingerling, Desirée, King Edward, Yukon Gold, Peruvian Purple, Pontiac

Best for Potato Salads and Scalloped Potatoes: Yellow Finn, Yukon Gold, new potato, red-skinned, white round, Peruvian Purple

Best for Mashing: Yukon Gold, russet, Peruvian Purple

Best for Soups: Yukon Gold, Yellow Finn, red-skinned, white round, Peruvian Purple

Best for Hash Browns: Red-skinned, white round, new potatoes, fingerling

Best for French Fries: Russet, Peruvian Purple, Desirée

Best for Potato Pancakes and Latkes: Russet, Yukon Gold

by color
Yellow Potatoes: With their creamy texture and buttery color and taste, yellow potatoes are truly multipurpose: great for roasting, baking, boiling, mashing, and steaming. Yukon Gold, Yellow Finn, and German Butterball are common yellow potatoes.

Red Potatoes: Red-skinned potatoes have white, yellow, or even red flesh. They are perfect for salads, roasting, grilling, boiling, and steaming and for making scalloped potatoes (see recipe in *The Vegan Table*), but not so good for mashed potatoes. Varieties include round red, Norland, Klondike Rose, and Pontiac.

Russet Potatoes: Also called Idaho, russets are high in starch and characterized by mottled brown skin and white flesh. Because they're light and fluffy when cooked, they're ideal for baking and mashing but not great for potato salads or scalloped potatoes.

White Potatoes: Considered an all-purpose potato, both round and long white potatoes are versatile and can be used in most potato preparations. White Rose, Kennebec, Superior, and Atlantic are examples of white potatoes.

Blue/Purple Potatoes: Originally from Peru, their flesh hues range from dark blue or lavender to white. They are good all-purpose potatoes that add drama to your dish. To retain their bright color, toss with lemon juice before and after cooking. Look for Russian Blue or Purple Viking.

Blueberry Croutons

▶ *Soy-free*

Enjoy these decadent little gems, especially during the summer months when blueberries are abundant and sweet.

1 cup (145 g) fresh ripe blueberries, picked through
½ cup (60 g) all-purpose flour
½ cup (120 ml) nondairy milk (such as almond, soy, rice, hazelnut, hemp, or oat)
1 cup (84 g) crushed cornflakes (pulsed in a coffee grinder or food processor)
2 to 3 tablespoons (30 to 45 ml) canola or grapeseed oil

compassionate cooks' tips

- This dish might require a little trial and error before you get it right. Working in small batches definitely helps, finding the right temperature of your burner is key, and staying close to the stove is essential.

- If your blueberries aren't super sweet or completely ripe, try adding a little sugar to the crushed cornflakes.

- 3 cups (84 g) whole cornflakes makes 1 cup (84 g) crushed. You don't want them completely pulsed into a powder because if you keep them textured you get some crisp when they're fried.

DIRECTIONS

Rinse the blueberries, shaking off the excess water but keeping them slightly wet and discarding any that are bruised or crushed.

Add the flour to a bowl, the milk to another bowl, and the crushed cornflakes to yet another.

Working in small batches (maybe 10 berries at a time), dip the blueberries into the flour and shake off the excess. Next dip the berries into the milk and then roll them in the cornflakes, coating them completely.

Heat the oil in a large sauté pan over medium-low heat. You don't want the heat so high that the berries will burst before the coating is crisp, and you don't want the coating to burn. Add the coated berries and fry until brown and crisp, gently shaking the pan to brown them evenly.

Transfer to a paper towel-lined plate and let cool before serving. Repeat until you've used all your blueberries.

YIELD: 8 servings, about 2 tablespoons (30 g) each

SERVING SUGGESTIONS AND VARIATIONS
- Add them to the Chilled Blueberry Mango Soup (page 140).
- Add them to a fresh spinach salad.
- Add a little sugar to the flour mixture and serve them as little dessert poppers.

PER SERVING: 112 Calories; 5g Fat (39.2% calories from fat); 2g Protein; 16g Carbohydrate; 1g Dietary Fiber; 0mg Cholesterol; 102mg Sodium.

German Red Cabbage (*Rotkohl*)

▶ *Soy-free if using soy-free Earth Balance, wheat-free*

A very common dish in Germany, *rotkohl* simply means "red cabbage."

1 medium head red cabbage, cored
   and finely shredded

2 large tart apples, peeled and sliced
   into matchsticks

1 large red onion, sliced

1 tablespoon (6 g) finely minced fresh ginger

1½ cups (355 ml) water

1 cup (235 ml) apple cider vinegar

½ cup (100 g) granulated or brown
   sugar (112 g)

1 tablespoon (14 g) nondairy butter
   (such as Earth Balance)

1 teaspoon (6 g) salt

6 whole peppercorns

2 whole allspice

2 whole cloves

2 bay leaves

1 tablespoon (8 g) cornstarch
   mixed with 1 tablespoon (15 ml)
   water (optional)

DIRECTIONS

Add the cabbage, apples, onion, and ginger to a large sauté pan, turn the heat to low, and stir to combine. Add the water, vinegar, sugar, butter, and salt. Add the peppercorns, allspice, cloves, and bay leaves to a spice bag (or make your own by placing them on a piece of cheesecloth and securing it with string to create a bag). Add this spice bag to the sauté pan.

Increase the heat and bring to a boil. Reduce the heat; cover and simmer for 1 hour and 15 minutes.

Discard the spice bag and serve as is, as a "warm winter slaw," as one of the testers defined it, or continue as directed below.

In a small bowl, stir the cornstarch and water until smooth. Add to the cabbage mixture. Bring to a boil; cook and stir for 1 to 2 minutes or until thickened. Serve hot or at room temperature as a side dish.

YIELD: 6 servings

SERVING SUGGESTIONS AND VARIATIONS

- Maple syrup may be used in place of the sugar.
- One of the brilliant testers for this recipe wondered if some teabags of chai tea wouldn't be a good replacement for the spice bags.
- Serve this as a side dish or as a topping for a hearty sandwich, such as one made with barbecued tofu or tempeh.

PER SERVING: 135 Calories; 3g Fat (15.6% calories from fat); 1g Protein; 30g Carbohydrate; 3g Dietary Fiber; 0mg Cholesterol; 400mg Sodium

compassionate cooks' tip

Although this dish smells pretty strong while it's cooking, it's actually milder than you might think. Trust the process and enjoy the outcome.

Eggplant with Sweet Miso (*Dengaku*) Sauce
▶ *Wheat-free*

I find that most dishes calling for eggplant use ridiculous amounts of oil. This can be easily remedied by steaming or baking the eggplant instead of frying it. This traditional Japanese sauce is one of my favorites and is so easy to prepare.

4 Japanese or Chinese eggplants (the long purple eggplants, NOT Italian globe eggplants)
1 tablespoon (15 ml) sesame oil, divided
¼ cup (60 ml) red or yellow/light miso
2 tablespoons (9 g) granulated sugar
¼ cup (60 ml) sake or white wine
3 to 4 tablespoons (24 to 32 g) sesame seeds, toasted

DIRECTIONS
Preheat the oven to 400°F (200°C, or gas mark 6).

Cut the eggplants in half, then lengthwise into ½-inch-wide x 2-inch-long (1.3 cm x 5 cm) strips.

Baste the eggplants with some of the sesame oil, and roast them in the preheated oven for 5 to 6 minutes, or place on a hot grill for 5 or 6 minutes.

Combine the miso, sugar, and sake in a small saucepan, and stir gently over low heat for 3 to 4 minutes or until the mixture starts to thicken. Remove from the heat and stir in the toasted seeds. Set aside.

Heat a nonstick sauté pan, add the remaining sesame oil, and then add the baked eggplant. Fry over medium heat until both sides are golden brown. Even though you've already cooked the eggplant, this step is just to add a little extra flavor. Don't overcook, or the eggplants may begin to fall apart.

Arrange the cooked eggplants on a serving plate and top with the sauce.

TOASTING SESAME SEEDS
Toast the seeds on your toaster oven tray or in an unoiled nonstick sauté pan over low heat, shaking the pan back and forth until the seeds start to pop and release an aromatic, toasted smell.

STEAMING THE EGGPLANT
Instead of baking the eggplant, you may also steam it in a simple steamer basket for about 10 minutes, making that last step of lightly frying the eggplant more necessary for adding flavor.

YIELD: 6 servings

PER SERVING: 177 Calories; 7g Fat (32.3% calories from fat); 6g Protein; 25g Carbohydrate; 9g Dietary Fiber; 0mg Cholesterol; 434mg Sodium

compassionate cooks' tip
Different brands of miso have various strengths and flavors; if you prepare this recipe as described but find the resulting dish too salty, add some more sugar to balance it out. Red miso is stronger than white, so if you'd prefer it to be more mild-tasting, use the latter.

Linguine with Purple Cabbage

▶ *Soy-free*

Long strands of linguine combine with long strands of garlic-flavored cabbage in this delicious albeit simple dish.

¼ cup (60 ml) olive oil

2 medium red onions, thinly sliced

6 large cloves garlic, minced

1 large head red cabbage, thinly sliced
   (8 cups [560 g])

1 pound (455 g) linguine

Salt and freshly ground pepper, to taste

½ cup (70 g) toasted pine nuts

compassionate cooks' tip

Salting the water before adding the pasta helps achieve the al dente texture, where it is chewy in the middle but not undercooked.

DIRECTIONS

In a large sauté pan, heat the olive oil. Add the sliced onions, cover, and cook over medium-low heat, stirring occasionally, until tender and glistening, about 10 minutes.

Add the garlic and cook for about 3 minutes longer, uncovered, stirring periodically. Add the cabbage, cover, and cook, stirring occasionally, until the cabbage is tender, about 20 minutes.

Meanwhile, in a large pot of boiling water, cook the linguine according to package directions until al dente ("to the tooth"). Drain the pasta, reserving 1 cup (235 ml) of the cooking water in a bowl or cup. Return the pasta to the empty pot.

Add the cabbage-onion mixture to the pasta in the pot. Pour in the reserved pasta cooking water and toss well to combine. Season with salt and pepper.

Transfer to bowls, sprinkle with the pine nuts, and serve.

YIELD: 4 servings

SERVING SUGGESTIONS AND VARIATIONS

• Pulse the toasted pine nuts in a food processor before mixing with the cabbage and pasta.

• Toasted walnuts, in place of the pine nuts, add an earthy flavor to the dish.

PER SERVING: 678 Calories; 23g Fat (29.4% calories from fat); 21g Protein; 104g Carbohydrate; 9g Dietary Fiber; 0mg Cholesterol; 31mg Sodium

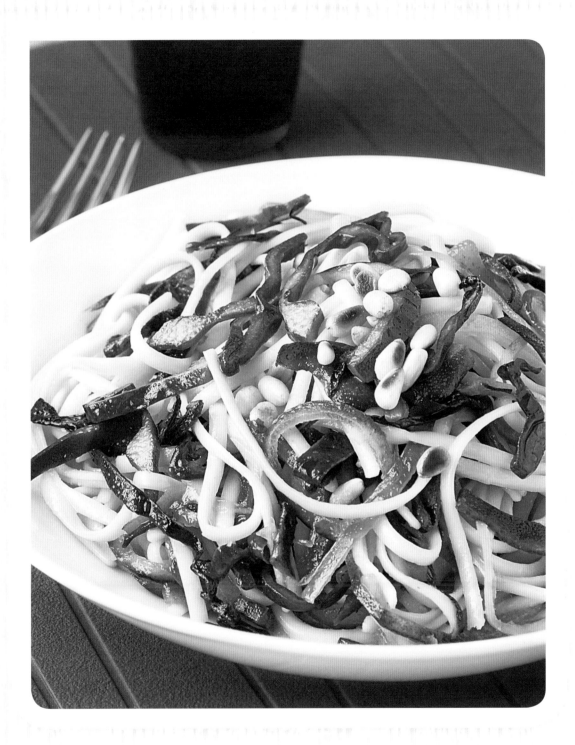

Potatoes and Eggplant (*Aloo Baingan*)

▶ *Wheat-free, soy-free*

This delicious main dish can be served with any bread or grain, or even as a sandwich filling on a hearty bun.

1 medium Italian globe purple eggplant, unpeeled, cut into ½-inch (1.3 cm) cubes

2 tablespoons (30 ml) canola oil, divided

1 teaspoon (2 g) cumin seeds

1 jalapeño pepper, minced

2 large yellow potatoes, unpeeled and cut into ½-inch (1.3 cm) cubes

¼ cup (60 ml) water

1 teaspoon (2 g) minced fresh ginger

1 tablespoon (6 g) ground coriander

½ teaspoon turmeric

½ teaspoon paprika

1 teaspoon (6 g) salt, to taste

4 medium tomatoes, diced

2 tablespoons (2 g) chopped cilantro or (8 g) parsley

DIRECTIONS

In a steamer basket on the stove top, steam the eggplant cubes until tender, about 15 minutes.

Add 1 tablespoon (15 ml) of the oil to a large sauté pan and heat over medium heat. Add the cumin seeds and fry until they begin to pop, watching closely and stirring frequently to prevent burning. Add the chile pepper and cook for about 5 minutes.

Add the potatoes, water, ginger, coriander, turmeric, paprika, and salt. Cover and sauté until they are cooked through, about 20 minutes, stirring occasionally to prevent sticking. I also add a little extra oil or water, if necessary.

Add the steamed eggplant and tomatoes and stir to coat. Cook for about 5 minutes longer until all the vegetables are heated through and thoroughly coated with the spices.

At the very end of cooking, add the chopped cilantro and mix well. Serve hot over brown rice or any preferred cooked grain.

YIELD: 4 servings

PER SERVING: 187 Calories; 8g Fat (35.6% calories from fat); 5g Protein; 28g Carbohydrate; 6g Dietary Fiber; 0mg Cholesterol; 602mg Sodium

Blueberry Buckle

▶ *Soy-free (depending on the milk and yogurt used)*

In my first cookbook, *The Joy of Vegan Baking*, I included cobblers, crisps, and crumbles and thought it was time to add a "buckle" to the list of these fairly similar desserts. The main difference has to do with the topping variations (biscuit crust in the case of cobblers, crumb/nut/oatmeal topping for crumbles and crisps).

¾ cup (150 g) granulated sugar

½ cup (112 g) nondairy butter (such as Earth Balance), softened, divided

1 container (6 ounces, or 170 g) nondairy yogurt (plain, vanilla, or even blueberry)

2 ⅓ cups (280 g) all-purpose flour, divided

2 teaspoons (5 g) baking powder

½ teaspoon salt

½ cup (120 ml) nondairy milk (such as almond, soy, rice, hazelnut, hemp, or oat)

¼ cup (60 ml) orange, apple, or pineapple juice

2 cups (290 g) fresh blueberries, rinsed and picked through

½ cup (115 g) firmly packed light brown sugar

½ teaspoon ground cinnamon

DIRECTIONS

Preheat the oven to 375°F (190°C, or gas mark 5). Lightly oil an 8 x 8-inch (20 x 20 cm) pan.

In a large bowl, cream together the sugar, ¼ cup (60 g) of the nondairy butter, and yogurt.

In a separate bowl, combine 2 cups (240 g) of the flour, baking powder, and salt. Add to the sugar/butter mixture, along with the milk and juice. Stir to combine and then fold in the blueberries. Pour into the prepared pan. (It's okay if the batter is thick.)

To make the streusel topping, combine the brown sugar, remaining ⅓ cup (40 g) flour, cinnamon, and remaining ¼ cup (60 g) butter. Distribute evenly over the cake batter.

Bake for 35 to 45 minutes or until a toothpick inserted into the center of the cake comes out clean.

YIELD: 10 to 12 servings

PER SERVING: 264 Calories; 8g Fat (26.0% calories from fat); 3g Protein; 46g Carbohydrate; 2g Dietary Fiber; 0mg Cholesterol; 142mg Sodium

food lore

The "buckle," which is usually made with blueberries, is similar to a crumble in that it has a streusel topping, but the main layer is actually a cake with the berries baked right into it, as opposed to a loose berry/sugar combination characteristic of the crumble. It may remind you of what is traditionally called a "coffee cake."

The "buckle" is called such because as it bakes, it rises unevenly, or "buckles," caused by the weight of the streusel on top.

Blackberry Breakfast Bars

▶ *Soy-free if using soy-free Earth Balance*

A delicious snack, breakfast, or dessert, these bars may be served on their own or with some nondairy yogurt. One tester described them as a cross between a breakfast bar and a mini cobbler.

2 cups (290 g) blackberries or raspberries (or a combination of each type), rinsed

2 tablespoons (9 g) granulated sugar

2 tablespoons (30 ml) water

1 tablespoon (15 ml) fresh lemon juice

¾ teaspoon ground cinnamon, divided

1 cup (120 g) all-purpose or whole wheat pastry flour

1 cup (80 g) quick-cooking oats

⅔ cup (150 g) firmly packed light or dark brown sugar

¼ cup (28 g) ground flaxseed

⅛ teaspoon baking soda

½ cup (112 g) nondairy butter (such as Earth Balance), melted

compassionate cooks' tip

If you'd like, you may strain the berry mixture once it's cooked to remove the seeds.

DIRECTIONS

Preheat the oven to 350°F (180°C, or gas mark 4).

In a medium saucepan, combine the blackberries, sugar, water, lemon juice, and ½ teaspoon of the cinnamon. Cover and bring to a boil. Reduce the heat and remove the cover. Simmer, uncovered, for about 8 minutes, stirring frequently. The mixture may begin to thicken up a bit by this point. Remove from the heat and set aside.

In a medium bowl, combine the flour, oats, brown sugar, ground flaxseed, the remaining ¼ teaspoon cinnamon, and the baking soda. Stir in the melted butter, and mix until thoroughly combined.

Press half of the flour-oat mixture into an ungreased 8 x 8-inch (20 x 20 cm) pan. (Set aside the other half to use as a topping.) Bake in the preheated oven for 20 to 25 minutes until the blackberries begin to bubble a bit. Remove from the oven.

Spread the berry mixture on top of the baked crust. Sprinkle with the reserved oat mixture and lightly press it into the berry filling.

Return to the oven for 20 minutes longer or until the topping turns a golden brown.

Cool in the pan on a wire rack. Cut into bars.

YIELD: 12 to 16 bars, depending on size

SERVING SUGGESTIONS AND VARIATIONS

Add chopped walnuts to the topping mixture.

PER SERVING: 151 Calories; 6g Fat (37.2% calories from fat); 2g Protein; 22g Carbohydrate; 2g Dietary Fiber; 0mg Cholesterol; 14mg Sodium

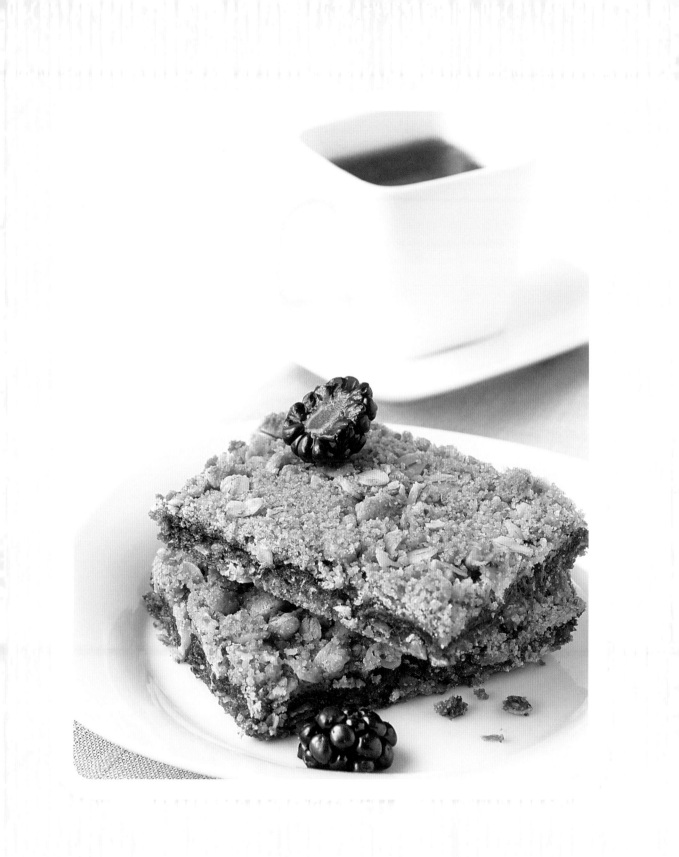

Quinoa Blue Cornbread

▶ *Soy-free, oil-free*

Thank my friend and colleague Cathy Fisher, chef and cooking instructor, for concocting this delicious, fat-free bread.

2 tablespoons (14 g) ground flaxseed (equivalent of 2 eggs)

1 cup plus 6 tablespoons (325 ml) water, divided

½ cup (25 g) uncooked quinoa

1 cup (140 g) blue cornmeal

½ cup (60 g) all-purpose or (60 g) whole wheat pastry flour

2 teaspoons (5 g) baking powder

1 teaspoon (3 g) baking soda

½ teaspoon sea salt

½ ripe banana

¾ cup (175 ml) nondairy milk (such as almond, soy, rice, hazelnut, hemp, or oat)

¼ cup (50 g) granulated sugar

1 cup (145 g) fresh blueberries or (154 g) corn kernels

DIRECTIONS

Preheat the oven to 350°F (180°C, or gas mark 4). Lightly oil an 8 x 8-inch (20 x 20 cm) or a 9 x 9-inch (23 x 23 cm) square cake pan.

In a food processor, blender, or in a bowl using an electric hand mixer, whip the flaxseed and 6 tablespoons (90 ml) of the water together until you have a thick and creamy consistency, 1 to 2 minutes.

Bring the remaining 1 cup (235 ml) water to a boil in a small saucepan and then add the dry quinoa. Reduce to a simmer, cover, and cook for 15 to 20 minutes until the water is gone and the quinoa is fluffy. (Add a little extra water if it evaporates before the quinoa is done.)

Meanwhile, in a medium bowl, combine the cornmeal, flour, baking powder, baking soda, and salt. In a separate bowl, mash the banana and combine it with the milk and sugar. Add the "flax eggs" and thoroughly combine.

Add the dry ingredients to the wet ingredients, along with the cooked quinoa, and stir to combine. Fold in the blueberries or corn kernels and stir just to combine. The mixture should be thick. Spread into the prepared pan and bake for 20 to 25 minutes until a toothpick inserted into the center comes out clean.

YIELD: 8 to 10 servings

PER SERVING: 134 Calories; 2g Fat (13.8% calories from fat); 3g Protein; 27g Carbohydrate; 2g Dietary Fiber; 0mg Cholesterol; 247mg Sodium

compassionate cooks' tip

Yellow cornmeal works just as well as blue, and according to Cathy, buckwheat flour gives the bread a nice earthy taste. Cathy also recommends any type of sugar, dry or liquid, including maple syrup or brown sugar.

WAYS TO INCREASE BLUE AND PURPLE FOODS

- Sprinkle frozen or fresh blueberries or blackberries on your cereal or oatmeal.

- Make coleslaw with shredded purple cabbage and purple carrots.

- Use purple potatoes in potato salad.

- Roast unpeeled purple and red potatoes with a drizzle of olive oil and a sprinkle of salt.

- Slice purple grapes and add to salads or eat whole as a snack.

- Use purple kale in a soup or stir-fry.

- Eat a plum or pluot for an afternoon snack and don't peel!

- Drink a glass of grape juice at breakfast.

- Add purple grapes to your morning smoothie.

- Make a salsa with blue corn and purple onions.

- Add a side of steamed purple asparagus, beans, or cauliflower at dinner.

- Eat a bowl of mixed berries for dessert, including blueberries, blackberries, and mulberries.

- Sprinkle raisins on top of a salad.

- Slice figs in half and drizzle on some agave nectar for a quick, healthful snack.

- Whip up a blueberry smoothie with banana, blueberries, and nondairy milk. (Add some peanut or almond butter for extra yumminess.)

Purple Plum Pie with Crumble Topping

▶ *Soy-free if using soy-free Earth Balance*

A perfect summer pie when plums (or pluots!) are sweet and ripe, this pie can be easily converted into a crumble or cobbler.

4 cups (900 g) sliced fresh plums or pluots, unpeeled

1 cup (200 g) granulated sugar, divided

¾ cup (90 g) all-purpose flour, divided

¼ teaspoon salt

¾ teaspoon ground cinnamon, divided

1 tablespoon (15 ml) lemon juice

1 (9-inch, or 23 cm) pie crust (homemade or store-bought)

½ cup (60 g) coarsely chopped walnuts

¼ teaspoon ground nutmeg

3 tablespoons (42 g) cold nondairy butter (such as Earth Balance)

DIRECTIONS

Preheat the oven to 375°F (190°C, or gas mark 5).

In a medium bowl, combine the plums, ½ cup (100 g) of the sugar, ¼ cup (30 g) of the flour, salt, ¼ teaspoon of the cinnamon, and lemon juice.

Pour into the pie crust and distribute evenly.

For the topping, combine the remaining ½ cup (100 g) sugar, remaining ½ cup (60 g) flour, walnuts, remaining ½ teaspoon cinnamon, and nutmeg in a small bowl. Cut in the nondairy butter and using your hands, mix until it resembles coarse crumbs. Sprinkle over the fruit.

Bake for 50 to 55 minutes or until bubbly and golden brown. Rotate once halfway through cooking to cook evenly and, if necessary, cover the edges of the crust during the last 20 minutes to prevent over-browning. Cool on a wire rack.

YIELD: 6 to 8 servings

SERVING SUGGESTIONS AND VARIATIONS

Instead of the crumble topping, you may make a covered pie, a cobbler, or a crisp.

PER SERVING: 379 Calories; 15g Fat (34.6% calories from fat); 5g Protein; 59g Carbohydrate; 3g Dietary Fiber; 0mg Cholesterol; 213mg Sodium

did you know?

A pluot is a cross between a plum and an apricot. It is my favorite stone fruit, particular the varieties called Flavor King and Flavor Supreme.

compassionate cooks' tips

- 8 plums or pluots will yield 4 cups (900 g) sliced.
- It's a good idea to add foil to the bottom rack of your oven to catch any drips.

Fresh Fig Upside-Down Cake

▶ *Soy-free if using soy-free Earth Balance and soy-free milk*

A wonderful way to use ripe figs, this cake is perfect for an autumnal feast.

¾ cup (170 g) nondairy butter (such as Earth Balance), divided

½ cup (115 g) firmly packed light brown sugar

2 tablespoons (30 g) agave nectar

10 to 12 fresh figs, stems removed, halved

1½ cups (180 g) unbleached all-purpose flour

1½ teaspoons (4 g) baking powder

¼ teaspoon salt

⅔ cup (130 g) granulated sugar

½ cup (125 g) silken tofu (firm)

¼ cup (60 ml) orange juice

¼ cup (60 ml) nondairy milk (such as almond, soy, rice, hemp, hazelnut, or oat)

1 teaspoon (5 ml) vanilla extract

compassionate cooks' tip

Fresh fig varieties include Brown Turkey, Sierra, and Black Mission.

DIRECTIONS

Heat the oven to 350°F (190°C, or gas mark 4). Lightly oil a 9-inch (23 cm) cake pan with 2-inch (5 cm) sides. Line the bottom of the pan with parchment paper and oil the parchment.

In a small saucepan over medium-low heat, melt ¼ cup (55 g) the nondairy butter. Stir in the brown sugar and agave nectar until smooth. Pour the sauce into the prepared cake pan. Arrange the figs, cut sides down, in concentric circles over the sauce. Set aside. In a medium bowl, combine the flour, baking powder, and salt. Set aside.

In a blender or food processor combine the granulated sugar, remaining ½ cup (115 g) butter, and silken tofu and process until smooth and thick. Add the orange juice, milk, and vanilla and process until thoroughly combined.

Add the tofu mixture to the dry ingredients and stir until just combined. The batter will be somewhat thick. Spoon it evenly over the figs.

Place the cake on the center rack and bake until golden brown and a toothpick inserted into the center comes out clean, 45 to 55 minutes. Transfer the cake to a rack and cool in the pan for at least 30 minutes.

Run a thin knife around the sides of the pan to loosen. Place a serving platter on top of the pan and invert the cake. Gently lift off the pan and remove the parchment paper.

YIELD: 8 to 10 servings

PER SERVING: 346 Calories; 14g Fat (35.1% calories from fat); 4g Protein; 54g Carbohydrate; 3g Dietary Fiber; 0mg Cholesterol; 103mg Sodium

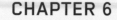
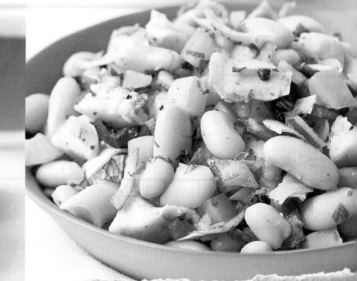

color me
WHITE/TaN

FIBER-RICH AND FILLING

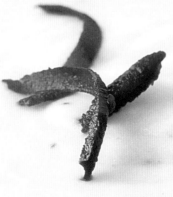
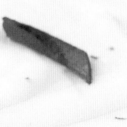

In a cookbook based on *color*, what role, you ask, do white and tan foods play? At a time when most people's meals are made up of drab-colored white and tan products (mostly in the form of starches, meat, dairy, and eggs), should we even include these light-hued foods in our spectrum? Although it's true that the more intensely colored the food is, the more healthful it is because of its health-promoting *pigments*, that doesn't mean white and tan plant foods don't have their place in a healthful diet. They do—big time.

All for Allicin

Perhaps the most frequently eaten white plant foods are garlic and onions, both of which are members of the allium family and both of which are rich in powerful sulfur-containing compounds that are responsible for their strong aromas as well as for many of their health-promoting effects (see "Taste the Onion Rainbow" on page 77 and "How to Chop Onions without Crying" on page 64). Other members of this family include leeks, scallions, chives, and shallots.

These members of the allium family emit a compound called *allicin* when the vegetable is chopped, crushed, or otherwise damaged in some manner. Think of it as the plant's own defense mechanism against bacteria, fungi, and insects. When "pests" break the surface by biting into it, for instance, or when we do the same by cutting into it, it releases its strong odor, acting as a natural deterrent.

These same antibacterial and antifungal properties benefit us when we consume it, but in order to fully utilize these enzymes, the vegetable *must not be* intact. It's essential for the cell walls to be broken. For this reason, some experts recommend crushing garlic, as an example, and letting it sit for 5 minutes before eating it. Some also suggest that raw, uncooked allium vegetables have the most benefit. Think of how the flavor and odor of garlic and onions are subdued by cooking; that's because the allicin isn't as strong.

But allium veggies are not the only white plant foods to boast healthful properties. Cauliflower, along with other cruciferous vegetables such as broccoli, Brussels sprouts, and kale, has high amounts of sulforaphane, which has been shown to have anticancer, antidiabetic, and antimicrobial effects. Parsnips abound in potassium, and coconuts contain high amounts of lauric acid, which has potent antiviral and antibacterial properties.

Fiber Abundance

And though all plant foods have fiber, those that are highest in fiber tend to fall into the white/tan spectrum, namely oats, oat bran, oatmeal, flaxseed, psyllium husks, walnuts, and wheat bran. In fact, grains, nuts, and beans—all rich in soluble and insoluble fiber—tend to be some variation of white, brown, or tan, thus fitting nicely into this chapter.

Egyptian Spice Mix (*Dukkah*)
▶ *Oil-free, soy-free, wheat-free*

This delicious combo of toasted nuts and seeds is a traditional staple in Egypt. It reminds me of a dish one of my neighbors brings to our annual National Night Out street parties, sprinkled on top of oil-brushed lavash or pita bread.

½ cup (75 g) hazelnuts
¼ cup (20 g) coriander seeds
3 tablespoons (24 g) sesame seeds
2 tablespoons (14 g) cumin seeds
1 tablespoon (5 g) black peppercorns
1 teaspoon fennel seeds
1 teaspoon dried mint leaves
½ teaspoon salt

compassionate cooks' tip

There is no need to peel the hazelnuts. The skin tends to slide off pretty easily once they're toasted and cooled, but it's not imperative that you remove it.

DIRECTIONS

To a heavy skillet over high heat or on a toaster oven tray, add the hazelnuts and dry-roast until slightly browned and fragrant, being careful not to burn. Remove from the heat and cool completely. Repeat the procedure with each of the seeds and the peppercorns, staying close by to avoid burning. Allow each of them to cool completely before proceeding.

Place the cooled nuts and seeds, along with the mint and salt, into a food processor and blend until the mixture is crushed. Do not allow the mixture to become a paste.

Store in an airtight container in a cool place for up to 1 month.

YIELD: 8 servings, about 2 tablespoons (30 g) each

SERVING SUGGESTIONS AND VARIATIONS

• Traditionally, dukkah is eaten by dipping fresh bread first into olive oil and then into the nut/seed mixture. It can also be sprinkled on salads or steamed or roasted vegetables.

• Use it as a seasoning for grilled, seared, or baked tofu or sprinkle it on a loaf of fresh bread, brushed with olive oil and baked in the oven at 350°F (180°C, or gas mark 4) for 20 minutes.

PER SERVING: 60 Calories; 5g Fat (66.1% calories from fat); 2g Protein; 4g Carbohydrate; trace Fiber; 0mg Cholesterol; 138 mg Sodium

Quinoa and Eggplant Caviar

▶ *Wheat-free*

This Peruvian grain (actually a seed) is becoming more popular in the United States and deservedly so. It's packed with protein, fiber, and loads of phytochemicals, and for our purposes here, it resembles caviar—but only in appearance! This is especially true if you can find black-colored quinoa.

1 small purple Italian globe eggplant

1 tablespoon (15 ml) olive oil

1 yellow onion, finely chopped

2 cloves garlic, minced

1 cup (50 g) uncooked quinoa

2 cups (470 ml) water or vegetable stock

3 tablespoons (3 g) minced fresh cilantro

3 tablespoons (12 g) fresh parsley, chopped

1½ tablespoons (23 ml) tamari soy sauce, or to taste

2 tablespoons (30 ml) fresh lemon juice, or to taste

Salt and freshly ground pepper, to taste

did you know?

Commercial caviar, which has driven many types of the sturgeon fish to be endangered, involves stunning the fish (usually by clubbing her on the head) and opening her up to extract her ovaries. Most caviar is harvested this way, though some "fish farmers" will first check the consistency of her eggs before killing her—by first making an incision in her abdomen, inserting a small tube, and sucking out a few eggs to test for color and consistency. If they're "just right," he'll kill her and harvest the caviar. If they're too "ripe"— if the fish has begun to break them down for reabsorption—he'll put her back in the water and wait until her next reproductive cycle.

DIRECTIONS

Preheat the oven to 400°F (200°C, or gas mark 6). With a fork or sharp knife, prick the eggplant or make incisions in several spots all over. Place on a lightly oiled baking sheet and roast for 45 minutes to 1 hour or until soft and wrinkled.

Meanwhile, heat the olive oil in a large sauté or saucepan with a lid. Add the onion and garlic and cook over medium heat until the onion is soft and slightly golden brown, about 7 minutes.

Stir in the quinoa and lightly toast for 1 minute. Stir in the water, and bring to a boil. Reduce the heat, cover the pan, and gently simmer for 15 minutes.

Remove the pan from the heat and let stand for 10 minutes. Uncover the pan and fluff the quinoa with a fork. Transfer to a mixing bowl and let cool.

When the eggplant is cool enough to handle, peel off the skin and compost it. Place the flesh of the eggplant in a food processor with the cilantro, parsley, tamari, and lemon juice. Purée to a smooth paste and season with salt and pepper to taste.

Stir the eggplant mixture into the quinoa. Adjust the seasonings, adding tamari, pepper, or lemon juice to taste. Let it sit for about 15 minutes before serving to let the flavors and textures mingle.

YIELD: 4 to 6 servings

PER SERVING: 92 Calories; 3g Fat (30.3% calories from fat); 2g Protein; 15g Carbohydrate; 3g Dietary Fiber; 0mg Cholesterol; 402mg Sodium

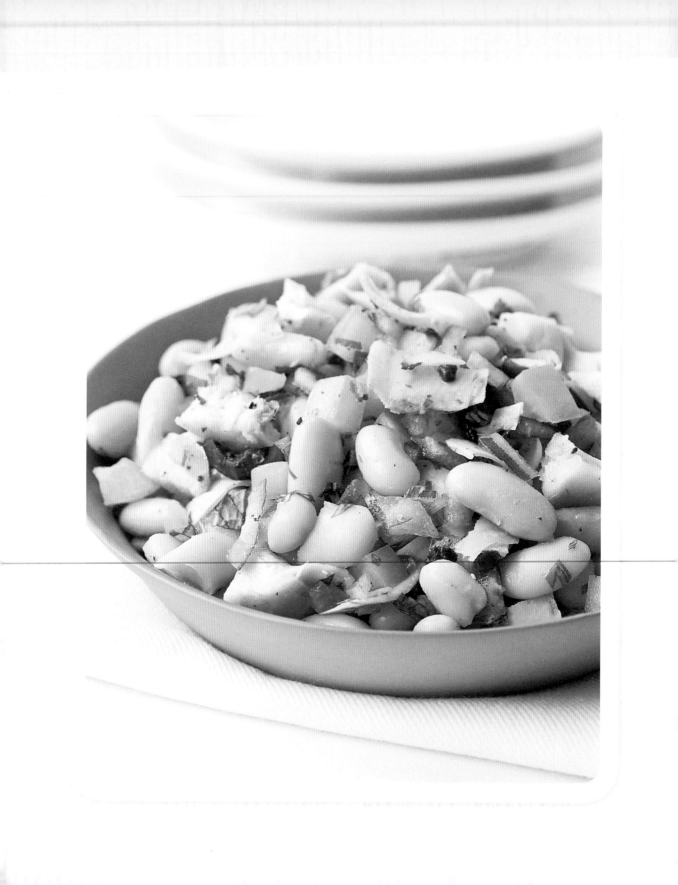

advance preparation required

White Bean and Artichoke Salad

▶ *Soy-free, wheat-free*

I love simple bean/veggie/herb salads such as this one.

2 cans (15 ounces, or 420 g) white beans, drained and rinsed

½ or 1 can (14 ounces, or 395 g) artichoke hearts, drained and roughly chopped

1 red, orange, or yellow bell pepper, diced

⅓ cup (33 g) pitted black olives, finely chopped

1 small red onion, finely chopped

¼ cup (16 g) chopped fresh parsley

¼ cup (16 g) chopped fresh mint leaves

2 tablespoons (8 g) chopped fresh basil

¼ cup (60 ml) olive oil

¼ cup (60 ml) red wine or balsamic vinegar

Salt and freshly ground pepper, to taste

DIRECTIONS

In a large bowl, combine the beans, artichoke hearts, bell pepper, olives, onion, parsley, mint, and basil.

In a jar or small bowl, combine the oil and vinegar; shake together or mix well. Pour the oil and vinegar over the salad and toss to coat. Season with salt and pepper.

Cover and chill in the refrigerator for several hours or overnight, stirring occasionally, to let the flavors blend.

YIELD: 6 servings

SERVING SUGGESTIONS AND VARIATIONS

• Use hearts of palm in place of artichoke hearts.
• The type of white bean you use is up to you, just try to keep it around 3 cups (420 g). Cannellini beans are simply white kidney beans, so they're hearty and large. Great Northern are smaller than cannellini but larger than navy beans, also called haricot, which are on the smaller side.

PER SERVING: 213 Calories; 10g Fat (41.4% calories from fat); 7g Protein; 24g Carbohydrate; 5g Dietary Fiber; 0mg Cholesterol; 220mg Sodium

Spicy Indian Garlic Relish

▶ *Soy-free, wheat-free*

This delicious condiment utilizes all the primary flavors of Indian cuisine: spicy, sweet, salty, and tart.

¼ cup (60 ml) canola or grapeseed oil

1 tablespoon (11 g) whole mustard seeds

1½ cups (204 g) peeled whole cloves garlic

2 teaspoons ground coriander

1 teaspoon ground cumin

1 teaspoon crushed red pepper flakes

½ teaspoon turmeric

1 teaspoon salt

2 tablespoons (30 g) dark brown sugar

¼ cup (60 ml) rice or apple cider vinegar

compassionate cooks' tip

Because the vinegar preserves the garlic, this is something you can store in a jar in the fridge for up to 4 weeks.

DIRECTIONS

Place the oil and mustard seeds in a sauté pan over medium heat. When the seeds begin to pop, stir them around a bit so they don't burn. You may also place a splatter screen on top of the pan or use a makeshift version by placing a cooling rack with a paper towel over the pan. Do not use a lid. It will trap moisture, which is not what you want.

After the seeds have been popping for about a minute, add the garlic cloves and cook for about 5 minutes until they start browning around the edges.

Add the coriander, cumin, red pepper flakes, turmeric, and salt and stir to combine with the garlic cloves. Cook for 1 to 2 minutes then add the brown sugar and vinegar. Bring to a boil, stir, and turn off the heat. Serve warm or cooled.

YIELD: 10 servings, about 2 tablespoons (30 g) each

SERVING SUGGESTIONS AND VARIATIONS

Serve as marinade or spread. Use as a condiment for Indian cuisine and with Indian breads.

PER SERVING: 99 Calories; 6g Fat (51.9% calories from fat); 2g Protein; 11g Carbohydrate; 1g Dietary Fiber; 0mg Cholesterol; 219mg Sodium

Parsnip Soup

▶ *Oil-free, wheat-free*

An underused root vegetable related to the carrot, parsnips have been eaten since ancient times. They pair well with the miso in this creamy, autumnal soup inspired by a similar recipe in *The Millennium Cookbook*.

2 yellow onions, roughly chopped

4 parsnips, peeled and chopped into uniform-size pieces

1 large yellow potato, peeled and diced

2 teaspoons minced garlic

1 teaspoon minced fresh ginger

⅓ cup (80 ml) dry white wine or non-alcoholic white wine

¼ teaspoon salt, plus more to taste

1 bay leaf

1 teaspoon dried thyme

1 teaspoon dried tarragon

¼ teaspoon ground nutmeg

2 cups (470 ml) vegetable stock

⅓ cup (83 g) yellow/light miso

4 cups (940 ml) nondairy milk (such as almond, soy, rice, hazelnut, hemp, or oat)

Freshly ground pepper, to taste

DIRECTIONS

In a large soup pot, combine the onions, parsnips, potato, garlic, ginger, wine, and salt. Cook over medium heat for 10 minutes or until the liquid evaporates.

Add the bay leaf, thyme, tarragon, nutmeg, and stock. Cover and simmer for 30 to 40 minutes or until the parsnips are fork-tender.

Once the parsnips are tender, remove the bay leaf, transfer the soup to a blender or food processor, and add the miso. Blend until smooth. Return to the pot and stir in the milk. Add salt and pepper to taste, rewarming the soup over low heat. Do not bring to a boil.

Ladle the soup into individual serving bowls. Serve hot, garnished with the suggestions below.

YIELD: 4 servings

SERVING SUGGESTIONS AND VARIATIONS

• Serve the soup topped with beautiful carrot curls. Using a vegetable peeler, create long, thin carrot strips from one carrot. Fry them in a little olive oil and salt until they are crispy, brightly colored, and even a little charred. Place on a paper towel to soak up any excess oil.

• Instead of carrot curls, try toasted pumpkin seeds, which add color, texture, crunch, and extra nutrients.

PER SERVING: 237 Calories; 1g Fat (3.0% calories from fat); 4g Protein; 53g Carbohydrate; 13g Dietary Fiber; 0mg Cholesterol; 160mg Sodium

compassionate cooks' tips

• Feel free to use an unsweetened milk for this soup (and others). Many plant-based milks have unsweetened counterparts.

• When shopping for parsnips, use the same criteria you would for carrots. Choose small, medium, or large but just make sure they are firm and not limp.

Roasted Garlic Soup

▶ *Wheat-free, soy-free is using soy-free milk*

I suppose if I had to pick two vegetables I couldn't live without, garlic would be one (kale would be the other). Raw, roasted, sautéed, or pickled, garlic is something I just can't get enough of. Considering how much garlic is in this soup, I hope you feel the same way!

4 large heads/bulbs garlic

¼ cup (60 ml) olive oil

1 tablespoon (15 ml) water or oil, for sautéing

1 leek, chopped

1 yellow onion, chopped

2 medium yellow potatoes, peeled and cubed

4 cups (940 ml) vegetable stock

⅓ cup (80 ml) dry white wine

¼ cup (60 ml) nondairy milk (such as almond, soy, rice, hazelnut, hemp, or oat)

1 tablespoon (15 ml) lemon juice, or to taste

Salt and freshly ground pepper, to taste

2 tablespoons (6 g) chopped fresh chives, for garnish

DIRECTIONS

Preheat the oven to 350°F (180°C, or gas mark 4).

Cut off the top ¼ inch (6 mm) of each garlic head to expose some of the actual garlic cloves. (The top of the garlic is the pointy part.) Place in a small, shallow baking dish (cut side up) and drizzle with the olive oil. Bake until the skins of the heads are golden and the garlic cloves themselves are soft, about 1 hour. Cool slightly. Press the individual garlic cloves between your thumb and finger to release. Although they are buttery soft at this point, just give them a little chop and set aside.

Heat the water in a large saucepan over medium heat. Add the roasted garlic cloves, leek, and onion and sauté until the onion is translucent, about 7 minutes. Add the cubed potatoes, stock, and white wine. Simmer over low-medium heat for 20 to 25 minutes until the potatoes are fork-tender.

Transfer the soup to a blender or food processor, and purée until smooth.

Return the soup to the soup pot and add the milk. Simmer (but don't boil) for about 5 minutes or until hot. Add the lemon juice, to taste, and season with salt and pepper. Ladle into bowls. Garnish with the chives.

YIELD: 4 to 6 servings

PER SERVING: 295 Calories; 11g Fat (31.5% calories from fat); 8g Protein; 45g Carbohydrate; 3g Dietary Fiber; 0mg Cholesterol; 683mg Sodium

compassionate cooks' tip

To wash and chop a leek, cut the root off the leek, slice the leek in half crosswise, and cut away and discard the darkest green part. (The white part is more tender; the dark green is tougher.) Make 4 lengthwise cuts in the remaining portion of the leek. Wash the cut parts and outer layer of the leek under cold running water. Place the leek on a clean cutting board and carefully slice the leek crosswise into your desired size.

Miso Fennel Ginger Soup

▶ *Wheat-free*

One of my favorite soups in my own repertoire, this delicious combination heals what ails and can be whipped up in a matter of minutes.

1 tablespoon (15 ml) oil or nondairy butter (such as Earth Balance)
1 fennel bulb, trimmed, cored, and sliced
1 red onion, sliced
3 tablespoons (18 g) minced fresh ginger
2 tablespoons (32 g) yellow/light miso
1 tablespoon (16 g) red miso
4 cups (940 ml) vegetable stock
½ cup (50 g) cubed extra-firm tofu (optional)
Chopped scallions or chives, for garnish

compassionate cooks' tip

I recommend keeping miso as a staple in the refrigerator to whip up quick soups, sauces, and dressings.

did you know?

Miso is produced by fermenting soybeans, rice, and/or barley. The taste varies according to the ingredients used, the temperature and duration of the fermentation process, and the amount of salt. White and red miso pastes are the most common, the former being milder than the latter.

DIRECTIONS

Heat the olive oil in a 3-quart (3 L) saucepan over medium-low heat and then add the fennel, red onion, and ginger; sauté until the veggies are translucent, about 7 minutes.

Meanwhile, in a bowl or measuring cup, add the miso pastes and a small amount of water and stir to thin out.

Add the stock to the onion/fennel mixture and stir the miso into the soup, making sure it is dissolved and fully combined with the broth. Heat for 10 minutes, but do not boil. Add the tofu cubes. Cook for another 5 minutes or so, remove from the heat, and serve hot, garnished with scallions.

YIELD: 4 servings

SERVING SUGGESTIONS AND VARIATIONS

- The broth itself is a great base for a noodle soup. You could even add cooked soba noodles at the very end of the cooking time.
- I cannot tell a lie; I even add greens to this soup (I'm a greens junkie and add them to everything I can). A half-bunch of chopped-up chard or kale added toward the end of cooking time rounds out the soup.
- At times when I've had only stronger-tasting red miso in the house, I definitely use a lot less than I would the more mild-tasting yellow/light. Try 1 tablespoon (16 g) and then another until you have the taste you prefer.

PER SERVING: 107 Calories; 6g Fat (48.4% calories from fat); 3g Protein; 11g Carbohydrate; 2g Dietary Fiber; 0mg Cholesterol; 1445mg Sodium

Winter White Soup

▶ *Wheat-free, soy-free if using soy-free milk, oil-free if sautéing in water*

The name alone evokes a chilly night with the fire blazing, romance swirling, and kitties purring on my lap. At least, that's where you'll find me when enjoying this soup!

1 tablespoon (15 ml) oil or water, for sautéing

3 cloves garlic, chopped

2 shallots, chopped

1 (1-inch, or 2.5 cm) piece fresh ginger, minced

3 scallions, chopped

3 yellow potatoes, peeled and cubed

2 medium parsnips, chopped

1 apple or pear, peeled and cubed

1 can (15 ounces, or 420 g) white beans, drained and rinsed

1 teaspoon chopped fresh dill

1 teaspoon dried tarragon

¾ cup (180 ml) dry white wine

6 whole sprigs fresh thyme

3 cups (705 ml) vegetable stock

¼ cup (60 ml) nondairy milk (such as almond, soy, rice, hemp, hazelnut, or oat)

Salt and freshly ground pepper, to taste

Grated red beet, for garnish

DIRECTIONS

Heat the oil in a soup pot over medium-low heat. Add the garlic, shallots, ginger, and scallions and cook until fragrant but not brown, about 5 minutes.

Add the potatoes, parsnips, apple, beans, dill, and tarragon and cook for 5 minutes longer, stirring occasionally.

Stir in the wine and thyme and turn up the heat to high. Boil, stirring constantly, until the wine is reduced by half, about 5 minutes. Pour in the vegetable stock. Return the mixture to a boil, then reduce the heat to low and simmer, partly covered, until the vegetables are tender, about 20 minutes.

Remove the thyme sprigs and transfer to a blender. Purée until smooth, working in batches if necessary. Alternatively, you may use an immersion blender and purée the soup right in the soup pot after removing the thyme sprigs.

Stir in the milk, season with salt and pepper, and top with the grated red beet, for garnish. The red contrasts beautifully with the white soup. Serve hot.

YIELD: 4 servings

PER SERVING: 410 Calories; 5g Fat (12.2% calories from fat); 12g Protein; 75g Carbohydrate; 14g Dietary Fiber; 0mg Cholesterol; 769mg Sodium

compassionate cooks' tip

Any white bean works well, including Great Northern, cannellini, or navy.

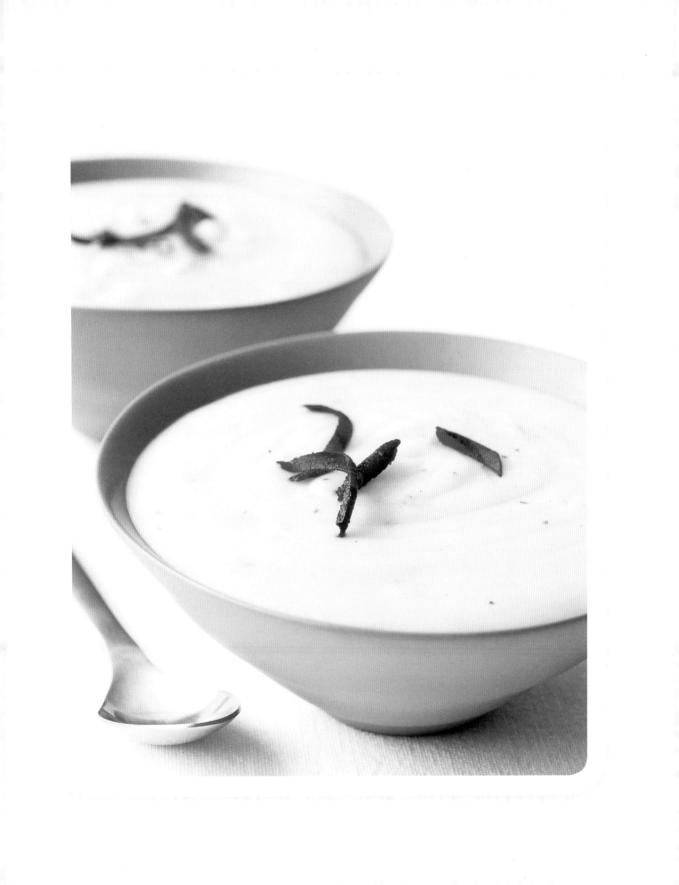

Quinoa, Tofu, and Kale with Walnut Pesto

▶ *Wheat-free*

I made this for a Labor Day party along with several other dishes, and this was my absolute favorite. Featuring some of my favorite foods, this is a great make-ahead dish that yields a large amount.

2 cups (100 g) uncooked quinoa

4 cups (940 ml) water or vegetable stock

2 tablespoons (30 ml) olive oil, divided

1 block (10 or 12 ounces, or 280 or 340 g) extra-firm tofu, cubed

1 bunch kale, finely chopped

⅓ cup (40 g) toasted pumpkin seeds

¼ cup (28 g) finely chopped sun-dried tomatoes, oil-packed or dried and reconstituted

Salt and freshly ground pepper, to taste

⅓ cup (85 g) Walnut Basil Pesto (page 108)

DIRECTIONS

Using a fine mesh strainer, rinse the quinoa under running water.

Next, add the rinsed quinoa along with the water to a 3-quart (3 L) saucepan. Cover and bring to a boil over medium heat. Reduce the heat to medium-low and cook until the quinoa absorbs all the water and fluffs up, about 15 minutes. Turn off the heat and keep covered.

Meanwhile, heat up 1 tablespoon (15 ml) of the olive oil in a large sauté pan over medium heat. Sauté the tofu until golden brown on all sides, 10 to 12 minutes. Remove from the pan and transfer to a large bowl.

Add the remaining 1 tablespoon (15 ml) olive oil to the pan, and sauté the kale until tender and bright green, about 5 minutes. Add to the bowl with the tofu.

When the quinoa is cooked and cooled, add it to the bowl, along with the toasted pumpkin seeds, sun-dried tomatoes, salt and pepper to taste, and pesto. Mix well to fully incorporate the pesto. Serve right away or store in the fridge until ready to serve. Bring to room temperature before serving.

YIELD: 6 to 8 servings

PER SERVING: 194 Calories; 12g Fat (55.2% calories from fat); 7g Protein; 16g Carbohydrate; 3g Dietary Fiber; 0mg Cholesterol; 574mg Sodium

compassionate cooks' tips

- When you're making a small grain like quinoa and want to prevent it from turning out sticky after it's cooked, try this trick. Once the quinoa is cooked to the desired texture, turn off the heat and leave it covered for 10 minutes. Then, lift up the cover and fluff with a fork.

- Quinoa is fully cooked when it is tender and you can see a "curlicue" in each grain.

- My favorite tofu is Wildwood's super firm. If you can't find it, just use the firmest tofu you know of or even use frozen and thawed tofu (see page 181).

Jicama Slaw

▶ *Wheat-free, soy-free, oil-free*

Pronounced HIC-a-ma, this white root vegetable native to Mexico is crispy and refreshing and a delicious addition to salads. One tester's fabulous recommendation was to just chop it up and serve with salsa, a healthier alternative to corn chips.

1 large jicama (about 2 pounds, or 905 g), peeled and cut into matchsticks

½ head napa cabbage, shredded

2 carrots, shredded

½ cup (120 ml) fresh lime juice

¼ cup (60 ml) rice vinegar, seasoned or regular

2 tablespoons (15 g) chili powder

2 tablespoons (40 g) agave nectar

Salt and freshly ground pepper, to taste

¼ cup (16 g) finely chopped fresh cilantro

compassionate cooks' tip

Seasoned rice vinegar is sweetened with sugar. Consider doing this before adding the agave. Try 1 tablespoon (15 ml) at a time until you find the right level of sweetness.

DIRECTIONS

Combine the jicama, cabbage, and carrots in a large bowl. Set aside.

In a separate bowl, whisk together the lime juice, rice vinegar, chili powder, and agave. Season to taste with salt and pepper. The dressing may be made a day in advance, covered, and kept refrigerated. Bring to room temperature before using.

When ready to serve, pour the dressing over the jicama mixture and toss to coat well. Allow the salad to sit at room temperature for 15 minutes before serving.

Sprinkle the cilantro on top or mix it in with the salad before serving.

YIELD: 6 servings

SERVING SUGGESTIONS AND VARIATIONS

- For a lemon/lime dressing, use ¼ cup (60 ml) lime juice and ¼ cup (60 ml) lemon juice.
- Use sliced apples in place of or in addition to the jicama.
- Serve this slaw within a few hours of preparing it; it doesn't hold very well in the refrigerator overnight. You could always prepare it in advance by keeping the vegetables separate from the dressing until you're ready to serve.

PER SERVING: 105 Calories; 1g Fat (4.9% calories from fat); 2g Protein; 26g Carbohydrate; 9g Dietary Fiber; 0mg Cholesterol; 42mg Sodium

Coconut Rice

▶ *Soy-free, oil-free, wheat-free*

The aroma of the cooking rice will have you anxious with anticipation, and the flavor will inspire you to squeal with delight! Serve with Asian-style dishes and stir-fries, including the Quick Curried Swiss Chard on page 32.

1 can (15 ounces, or 420 g) light coconut milk

1¼ cups (295 ml) water

1½ cups (285 g) uncooked brown or jasmine rice

1 teaspoon coconut extract

1 teaspoon salt, or to taste

3 tablespoons (13 g) unsweetened coconut flakes (optional)

DIRECTIONS

In a saucepan, combine the coconut milk, water, rice, and coconut extract. Bring to a boil over medium heat. Cover, reduce the heat to low, and simmer for 40 minutes or until the rice is tender. (Check halfway through the cooking time and close to the end of the cooking time in case the liquid has evaporated and extra needs to be added.)

Turn off the heat and let sit, covered, for 5 minutes. Remove the lid and fluff with a fork. Season with salt to taste and add the coconut flakes, if using. Stir to combine and serve.

YIELD: 4 servings

PER SERVING: 340 Calories; 9g Fat (23.6% calories from fat); 7g Protein; 58g Carbohydrate; 1g Dietary Fiber; 0mg Cholesterol; 566mg Sodium

did you know?

To produce brown rice, only the outermost layer (the hull) is removed. To produce white rice, the bran and most of the germ layer is also removed, thus removing most of the nutrients, including the fiber. In the final processing stage, the rice is polished (to create a shiny white grain and to extend the shelf life of the product), thus removing the aleurone layer, which contains the essential fats. White rice, such as jasmine, is okay when you want to emphasize the white color, but in general, try to choose brown rice.

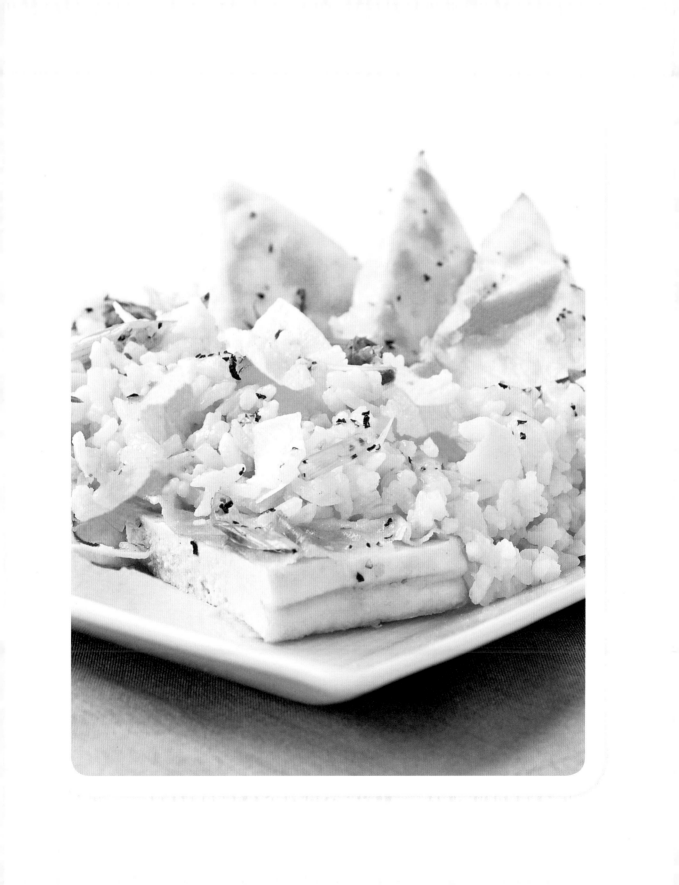

Roasted Fennel

▶ *Wheat-free, soy-free*

Normally, fennel tastes like a cross of celery, cabbage, and licorice. Roasting, however, deepens the flavor from the caramelizing. Add the gorgeous Carrot Purée (page 56), and you've got a great appetizer or side dish of sweet and savory flavors.

4 fennel bulbs
2 tablespoons (30 ml) olive oil
2 tablespoons (30 ml) balsamic vinegar
Salt and freshly ground pepper, to taste

DIRECTIONS

Preheat the oven to 400°F (200°C, or gas mark 6).

Cut off the stems of the fennel, slice the fennel in half lengthwise, place the cut side down, and cut into ½-inch (1.3 cm) slices. Toss on a baking sheet with enough olive oil and balsamic vinegar to coat and sprinkle with salt and pepper. Spread evenly on the baking sheet.

Roast for 25 to 30 minutes until tender, turning the slices after about 15 minutes.

YIELD: 16 servings

SERVING SUGGESTIONS AND VARIATIONS

• Add a dollop of Carrot Purée (see page 56) to each roasted slice and serve as a side dish or an appetizer.
• Called *finnochio* in Italian, fennel is delicious raw in salads, puréed in soups, or roasted with a drizzle of olive oil, salt, and pepper.

PER SERVING: 22 Calories; 2g Fat (66.6% calories from fat); trace Protein; 2g Carbohydrate; 1g Dietary Fiber; 0mg Cholesterol; 11mg Sodium

did you know?

Anethole is the phytonutrient in fennel that is largely responsible for the characteristic flavor and fragrance of fennel, anise, and licorice. More than that, it has been found to have potent antibacterial, anti-inflammatory, and anticancer properties. It is also an effective repellent against mosquitoes.

Lemony Pan-Fried Chickpeas with Chard

▶ *Soy-free, wheat-free*

Frankly, you can use any leafy green veggie you choose, but I find the chard pairs particularly well with chickpeas.

1 tablespoon (15 ml) olive oil
1 small yellow onion, diced
1 can (15 ounces, or 420 g) cooked chickpeas
1 bunch Swiss chard, chopped
1 small lemon
½ teaspoon salt, or to taste
Freshly ground pepper, to taste

did you know?

There are 15 grams of protein in 1 cup (240 g) of cooked chickpeas.

food lore

Chickpeas—also called garbanzo beans and *ceci* (Italian for chickpea) —are incredibly versatile and used in many cultures' cuisines, including Indian, Pakistani, Middle Eastern, Mediterranean, and others. Cultivated for more than 7,500 years, chickpeas were considered a staple food in ancient Rome and classical Greece.

DIRECTIONS

Heat the olive oil in a large sauté pan over medium-high heat. Add the onion and cook for 5 minutes, or until it begins to turn translucent. Add the chickpeas and sauté until they begin to turn golden brown, about 10 minutes.

Stir in the chard and cook until it begins to shrink down and become tender, 5 to 7 minutes.

Using a microplane or lemon zester, zest the lemon before you cut it and add it to the pan. Cut the lemon in half and squeeze in the juice of one half (be sure to avoid adding the pits). Stir to combine and taste. Add salt and pepper and more lemon juice, if desired, and stir once more to combine.

Serve right away or at room temperature.

YIELD: 4 servings

SERVING SUGGESTIONS AND VARIATIONS

Spinach is a good substitute for chard because it also becomes buttery soft when cooked.

PER SERVING: 217 Calories; 6g Fat (24.7% calories from fat); 10g Protein; 33g Carbohydrate; 4g Dietary Fiber; 0mg Cholesterol; 285mg Sodium

Salt-and-Pepper Tofu

▷ *Wheat-free*

Not only one of my favorite ways to eat tofu, this is a quick meal that whips up in no time!

2½ tablespoons (38 ml) oil, divided
12 ounces (340 g) extra-firm tofu, sliced
　　into strips
1 teaspoon freshly ground black pepper
½ teaspoon paprika (smoked paprika, if
　　you can find it)
¼ teaspoon salt, or to taste
3 scallions, sliced
2 cloves garlic, minced

compassionate cooks' tip

Check out Resources and Recommendations on page 252 for where you can find smoked paprika. It adds a delicious depth of flavor and smokiness to whatever dish you're making.

DIRECTIONS

In a large sauté pan, heat 2 tablespoons (30 ml) of the oil over medium-high heat. Add the tofu and fry until the strips are golden brown and crispy on both sides, about 15 minutes. Meanwhile, in a small bowl, combine the pepper, paprika, and salt. Set aside.

When the tofu is done, remove from the pan and add the remaining ½ tablespoon (8 ml) oil to the pan to continue sautéing. Add the scallions and garlic and stir-fry for about 1 minute. Return the tofu to the pan and add the combined seasonings. Toss the tofu in the spices to coat and remove from the heat. Serve alone or with any of the sauces recommended below. (Serve them as accompaniments or add them to the cooking tofu just before you remove it from the heat.)

YIELD: 2 servings

SERVING SUGGESTIONS AND VARIATIONS

• Serve with an orange/agave sauce: Combine equal parts hoisin sauce (a Chinese condiment found in the Asian section of the grocery store) and agave nectar (see Resources and Recommendations) and 2 tablespoons (10 g) orange zest.

• Serve with chili/soy sauce: Combine equal parts red chili sauce/hot sauce and tamari soy sauce. Add a little olive oil, if desire.

• Serve with scallion/ginger sauce: Combine ⅓ cup (80 ml) seasoned rice vinegar, ¼ cup (60 ml) tamari soy sauce, 1 tablespoon (15 g) brown sugar, 1 finely chopped scallion, and ¼ teaspoon chopped fresh ginger.

PER SERVING: 300 Calories; 26g Fat (73.1% calories from fat); 15g Protein; 7g Carbohydrate; 3g Dietary Fiber; 0mg Cholesterol; 283mg Sodium

FREEZING TOFU

One of my favorite ways to eat tofu is to freeze it first. You can do this with any variation of firm tofu (firm, extra firm, or super firm) that is packed in water. Once you arrive home from the grocery store, fresh tub of tofu in hand, instead of putting it in the refrigerator, put it in the freezer. Don't open it, don't drain the water, and don't fuss with it. Just put the entire package in the freezer. (For best results, I recommend you let it freeze for at least 24 hours and it can last in the freezer for up to 6 months.)

When you're ready to use it, take it out of the freezer and thaw it on the counter for a few hours. I find that it thaws best on the counter rather than in the fridge. I usually tuck it into a corner where it is not in direct sunlight and just leave it alone until it is completely thawed.

Now the magic begins.

Open the package, dump out the water, hold the block of tofu over a large bowl or the sink, and really squeeze out all the water. The tofu will literally be like a sponge, and tons of water will come pouring out after you've thawed it. Now it's ready to be eaten and/or cooked.

There are several advantages to freezing/thawing tofu:

1) Because you've squeezed out so much water from this water-based food, you make it very porous. In fact, all the pores will be visible to your naked eye. And all of these pores create room for another liquid—in particular, a marinade—to penetrate the tofu and create more flavor.

2) The other thing you've done is change the texture completely. Tofu already has great texture when it's really firm, but it's even chewier after having been frozen and thawed. Even I, a rabid tofu fan, prefer the texture of thawed tofu to the regular stuff. And I *love* the regular stuff.

Now that you've thawed it, there are several ways to prepare it:

- Cube it or crumble it and toss it into green salads. (Check out the Greek Spinach Salad on page 107, in which the thawed tofu plays the role of feta.)

- Crumble it and add it to bean chili or marinara sauce.

- Add it to a stir-fry.

- Grill it or broil it.

Note: Even though silken tofu (the kind that is sold in vacuum-packed boxes and is found in the nonrefrigerated section of the grocery store) is designated as "soft," "firm," and "extra firm," this is not the type of tofu I'm referring to. When I talk about "firm" tofu, I mean the fresh, water-based type in the refrigerator case. Frozen silken tofu will not produce the same results.

advance preparation required

Tofu (*Koyadofu*) Teriyaki

▶ *Wheat-free*

This dish requires a little advance preparation because you will want to use tofu that has been frozen and thawed. Although you can use regular tofu, it won't absorb the marinade as well.

2 packages (10 ounces, or 280 g) extra-firm tofu, frozen and thawed

3 cups (705 ml) vegetable stock (store-bought or homemade)

⅔ cup (160 ml) tamari soy sauce

¼ cup (50 g) granulated sugar

2 tablespoons (30 ml) toasted sesame oil, plus more for frying

food lore

Koyadofu or *kogori dofu* is tofu that has been frozen and thawed, resulting in a spongy texture and brownish color. It is great stewed in broths or anything where it can soak up the flavor of the sauce without breaking apart. Legend has it that a monk left some tofu outside overnight in freezing temperatures. The next morning, he thawed the frozen tofu. It's been a traditional way of preparing it ever since.

DIRECTIONS

Gently squeeze the thawed tofu over a bowl or sink to remove excess moisture and cut into ½-inch (1.3 cm)-thick slices.

In a saucepan, combine the stock, tamari, sugar, and 2 tablespoons (30 ml) sesame oil. Bring to a boil, add the tofu, and cook for 5 to 6 minutes over low heat. Turn off the heat and let sit for 30 minutes or overnight.

Remove the tofu from the sauce and gently squeeze out the liquid. Reserve the sauce.

Heat the additional sesame oil in a frying pan, add the tofu, and fry over low to medium heat for 2 minutes on each side until golden brown. Alternatively, you may cook the tofu for about 3 minutes on each side under the broiler.

Arrange the tofu on a plate, spoon a little extra teriyaki sauce over the tofu, and serve.

YIELD: 4 servings

PER SERVING: 211 Calories; 11g Fat (45.4% calories from fat); 7g Protein; 23g Carbohydrate; 1g Dietary Fiber; 0mg Cholesterol; 1413mg Sodium

compassionate cooks' tip

If Wildwood brand (www.wildwoodfoods.com) is available in your area, look for super firm, which is my favorite.

Cashew and Red Lentil Burgers

▶ *Soy-free*

Many people ask about grilling veggie burgers, and I always recommend using a special grill pan, particularly when it comes to softer burgers such as these.

2 cups (470 ml) water

1 cup (130 g) diced carrots (2 to 4 medium carrots)

½ cup (100 g) red lentils, rinsed and picked through

½ teaspoon salt, plus more to taste

1 cup (150 g) raw cashews

2 tablespoons (30 ml) oil, divided

1 medium onion, chopped

1 clove garlic, minced

1 tablespoon (6 g) curry powder

1 cup (115 g) bread crumbs (more may be needed)

Freshly ground pepper, to taste

6 (6-inch, or 15 cm) whole wheat pita breads

Lettuce, tomatoes, and eggless mayonnaise, for toppings

DIRECTIONS

Combine the water, carrots, lentils, and ½ teaspoon salt in a saucepan. Bring to a boil. Reduce the heat to low and then cover and simmer until the lentils are tender and broken down, 12 to 14 minutes. Drain in a colander, pressing out the excess liquid. Transfer to a bowl and cool to room temperature, about 20 minutes.

Meanwhile, toast the cashews in a small dry skillet over medium-low heat or in the toaster oven until golden and fragrant. Let cool completely.

Heat 1 tablespoon (15 ml) of the oil in a large sauté pan over medium heat. Add the onion and cook, stirring, until softened, about 7 minutes. Add the garlic and curry powder and cook, stirring, for 1 minute. Remove from the heat and let cool.

Place the cooled cashews in a food processor and pulse until finely chopped. Add the lentils and the onion mixture; pulse until the mixture is cohesive but still somewhat textured. Transfer to a bowl and add enough bread crumbs to create a consistency that enables you to form cohesive patties. Season with salt and pepper to taste. With moist hands, form the mixture into six ½-inch (1.3 cm)-thick patties.

Add the remaining 1 tablespoon (15 ml) oil (or more, if necessary) to a large sauté pan over medium heat and cook the patties until evenly browned and heated through, about 4 minutes per side.

Serve in warmed pitas along with lettuce, tomatoes, and eggless mayonnaise.

YIELD: 6 patties

PER SERVING: 445 Calories; 14g Fat (27.7% calories from fat); 16g Protein; 68g Carbohydrate; 10g Dietary Fiber; 0mg Cholesterol; 792mg Sodium

compassionate cooks' tips

- Sometimes a white foam forms on the top of the water when cooking lentils. If this happens, simply skim the surface and remove it.

- These burgers freeze very well.

advance preparation required

Coconut Tapioca Pudding

▶ *Soy-free, oil-free, wheat-free*

A starch extracted from the root of the cassava plant native to Brazil, tapioca is used worldwide as a thickening agent. In this pudding, the pearls pair beautifully with the rich, creamy coconut milk.

2 cans (15 ounces, or 420 g) coconut milk
¼ teaspoon salt
1 tablespoon (8 g) cornstarch
½ cup (88 g) tapioca pearls
⅓ cup (67 g) granulated sugar
1 teaspoon pure vanilla extract
½ teaspoon ground cinnamon
Shredded coconut, for topping

did you know?

People tend to shy away from coconut milk and oil because of the saturated fat. However, not all saturated fats are created equal. Although tropical oils do still contain saturated fat, it is molecularly different than the animal-based saturated fat and doesn't appear to have the same detrimental effect on our bodies. Now, that isn't license to drink vats of coconut oil, but it does mean that coconut fat can be a healthful part of our diets.

DIRECTIONS

In a saucepan, bring the coconut milk and salt to a boil over medium heat, stirring occasionally. Remove a few tablespoons (45 to 60 ml) of the milk and add it to a bowl along with the cornstarch. Stir until the cornstarch dissolves and return it to the pot.

Turn down the heat to medium-low and add the tapioca pearls and sugar. Simmer for 15 to 17 minutes, periodically stirring to prevent the balls from sticking to one another.

At the end of 15 to 17 minutes (or when the balls are translucent), turn off the heat and stir in the vanilla and cinnamon.

You may serve it warm (perfect for winter), though I find that once it chills in the fridge for about an hour, it sets up even more.

Serve in bowls with shredded coconut and some extra cinnamon sprinkled on top.

YIELD: 4 servings

SERVING SUGGESTIONS AND VARIATIONS

Add chopped fresh mango to each serving.

PER SERVING: 397 Calories; 25g Fat (54.6% calories from fat); 2g Protein; 44g Carbohydrate; 3g Dietary Fiber; 0mg Cholesterol; 150mg Sodium

compassionate cooks' tips

- This pudding tends to be served best within an hour of making it only because it thickens up a lot when it's in the fridge.

- "Light" coconut milk is not thick enough to produce the desired results.

advance preparation required

Oat Bread

▶ *Soy-free*

The addition of rolled oats and oat bran provide texture, fiber, and flavor to this simple bread recipe.

1 envelope (2¼ teaspoons, or 7 g) active dry yeast

2¼ cups (530 ml) warm water

5 cups (625 g) all-purpose or whole wheat pastry flour

½ cup (40 g) rolled oats

¼ cup (25 g) oat bran

1 teaspoon salt

2 tablespoons (40 g) agave nectar or other liquid sweetener

2 tablespoons (30 ml) olive oil (optional)

DIRECTIONS

Add the yeast to the warm water, stir, and leave it to dissolve. Let it sit for 10 minutes. The yeast should begin to form a creamy foam on the surface of the water. If there is no foam, the yeast is dead and you should start over with a new packet. This process is called "proofing" to make sure the yeast is alive.

In a large mixing bowl (I use an electric stand mixer, but you can do it by hand), mix together the flour, oats, bran, and salt and make a well in the center. Pour the yeast and water mixture, agave nectar, and oil into the well. Stir from the center outward, incorporating the liquid ingredients into the flour. Mix until the mixture forms a soft dough. Add a small amount of water if the dough is too dry or a bit of flour if the dough is too sticky.

Turn out the dough onto a breadboard (or continue using the stand mixer). For best results, knead the dough for about 20 minutes without adding any more flour. If you're using a stand mixer, you won't need to do this for more than 10 minutes. The dough should be elastic and smooth. Place the dough in a lightly oil-coated bowl, cover with a damp cloth, and let sit in a warm, draft-free spot until doubled in size. At 70°F (21°C), this should take about 2½ hours.

After the allotted time, test the dough by poking a wet finger ½ inch (1.3 cm) into the dough. The dough is ready if the hole doesn't fill in. Gently press out the air, making the dough into a smooth ball. Return it to the bowl for a second rise, which will take about half as long as the first. Test with your finger after about 1 hour.

After the second rising, turn the dough out onto a lightly floured countertop or breadboard. Deflate the dough by pressing it gently from one side to the other. Cut it in half and form each part into a round ball. Let it rest, covered, for about 10 minutes.

Shape each ball into a loaf and place the loaves in one 9 x 5 x 3-inch (23 x 13 x 7.5 cm) or two 8 x 4 x 2-inch (20 x 10 x 5 cm) greased loaf pans. Let rise for about 30 minutes.

Preheat the oven to 425°F (220°C, or gas mark 7). Bake for 10 minutes, then lower the temperature to 325°F (170°C, or gas mark 3). Bake until they turn a golden brown color, 45 to 60 minutes. The loaves should slip easily out of the pans. When you tap their bottoms, they should sound hollow. Cool slightly before slicing.

YIELD: 2 loaves, about 24 slices/servings

PER SERVING: 121 Calories; 2g Fat (11.8% calories from fat); 3g Protein; 23g Carbohydrate; 1g Dietary Fiber; 0mg Cholesterol; 90mg Sodium

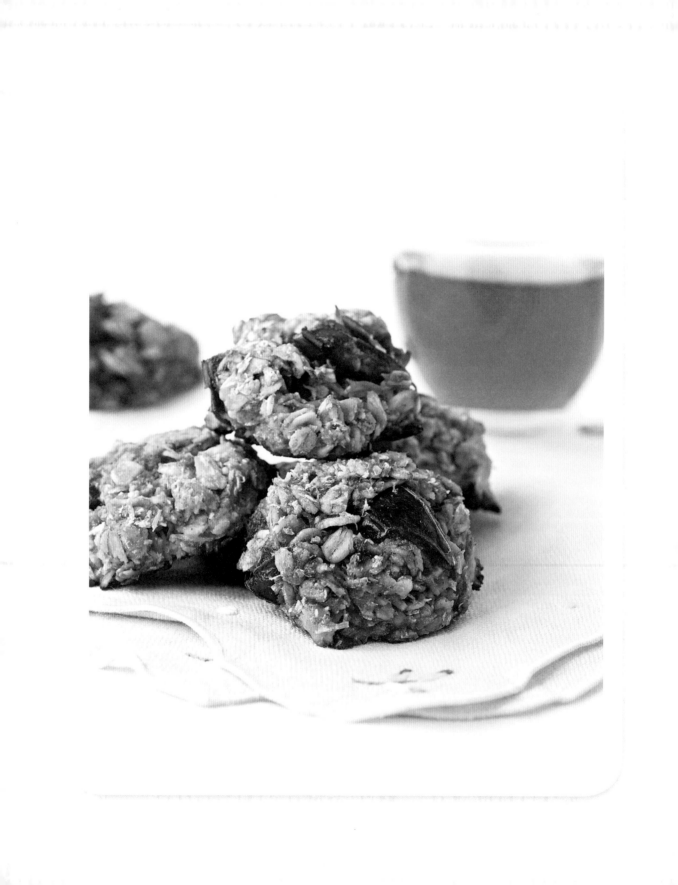

Banana Oat Date Cookies

▶ *Soy-free, wheat-free*

Children and adults alike love this incredibly healthful, delicious, sugar-free cookie that can be put together in no time and nibbled throughout the day.

3 large ripe bananas

1 teaspoon pure vanilla extract

¼ cup (60 ml) coconut butter or nondairy butter (such as Earth Balance), warmed until smooth

2 cups (160 g) rolled or quick-cooking oats

⅓ cup (23 g) unsweetened shredded coconut

½ teaspoon ground cinnamon

½ teaspoon salt

1 teaspoon baking powder

6 or 7 large dates, chopped (about ¼ cup, or 38 g)

DIRECTIONS

Preheat the oven to 350°F (180°C, or gas mark 4). Line 2 baking sheets with unbleached parchment paper.

In a large bowl, mash the bananas until smooth. Alternatively, you may purée them in a blender, though I like the lumpy texture when mashed by hand. Add the vanilla, coconut butter, oats, shredded coconut, cinnamon, salt, and baking powder and mix with your hands until fully combined. Fold in the chopped dates.

Drop dollops of the dough, each about 2 teaspoons in size, 1 inch (2.5 cm) apart, onto the prepared baking sheets. Press down a bit to flatten them. (They won't spread very much, so consider at this point what shape/size you want your finished cookies to be.) Bake for 15 minutes or until the cookies are golden brown on the bottom.

YIELD: 2 dozen cookies, or 24 servings

SERVING SUGGESTIONS AND VARIATIONS

- Add ½ cup (88 g) nondairy semisweet chocolate chips or a chopped-up dark chocolate bar at the same time you add the dates (or in place of them).
- If you have a hard time finding coconut butter, you may use the equivalent amount of any nut butter, such as peanut butter or almond butter, in its stead.
- One tester melted some nondairy semisweet chocolate chips and dipped half of each cookie into the chocolate and let it sit a bit before serving them.

PER SERVING: 61 Calories; 3g Fat (38.1% calories from fat); 1g Protein; 8g Carbohydrate; 1g Dietary Fiber; 0mg Cholesterol; 47mg Sodium

WAYS TO INCREASE WHITE AND TAN FOODS

- Choose brown rice—not white.

- Try different grains besides rice, such as quinoa, barley, or millet.

- Make a fruit salad using white nectarines and white peaches.

- Dip cauliflower into hummus for a snack.

- Add cauliflower florets to your salad.

- Roast garlic bulbs and spread on bread and vegetables instead of butter.

- Add crunchy jicama to your salad.

- Add minced shallots to your salad dressing.

- Include sliced onions and garlic cloves when roasting potatoes and other vegetables.

- Save your onion trimmings, including the papery brown skin, and store in the freezer in a well-sealed plastic freezer bag to add to soup stock.

- Experiment with the less common root vegetables, such as turnips, parsnips, daikon, celeriac, and kohlrabi.

- When stir-frying vegetables, start by sautéing generous quantities of finely chopped fresh ginger and garlic.

- Add minced scallions as a garnish to soups.

- For maximum phytochemical benefits, add raw garlic to salads and dressings.

- Add sliced pears to a spinach or green salad.

- Try a variety of onions. (See "Taste the Onion Rainbow" on page 77.)

- Make hummus from chickpeas or white beans and eat as a spread or dip.

- Add white beans to pasta sauce and salads.

- Add raw sweet onions to salads.

- Make oatmeal a regular breakfast item. I don't recommend instant oatmeal, but quick-cooking oats are a good alternative and cook up just as quickly when you add boiling water. They can be found in the bulk section of a natural grocery store and enable you to add your own flavorings and fruit. Although they take longer to cook, rolled oats and steel-cut oats are also very good options.

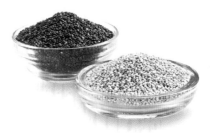

Sugar-and-Spice Almonds

▶ *Soy-free, wheat-free*

These almonds should come with a warning about how good they are. Fight the urge to eat them all in one sitting. Good luck.

¼ cup (50 g) granulated sugar

2 tablespoons (30 ml) oil (see tip below)

1 teaspoon cayenne pepper

½ teaspoon garlic salt (or sea salt)

½ teaspoon chili powder

¼ teaspoon crushed red pepper flakes

2 cups (290 g) unblanched whole almonds

DIRECTIONS

Preheat the oven to 250°F (120°C, or gas mark ½).

In a bowl, combine the sugar, oil, cayenne pepper, salt, chili powder, and red pepper flakes. Add the almonds and toss to coat thoroughly.

Spread in a single layer on a baking sheet and bake for 30 minutes or until lightly browned, stirring occasionally. Cool completely before storing in an airtight container.

YIELD: 8 servings, about ¼ cup (35 g) each

PER SERVING: 270 Calories; 22g Fat (70.4% calories from fat); 7g Protein; 14g Carbohydrate; 4g Dietary Fiber; 0mg Cholesterol; 134mg Sodium

compassionate cooks' tip

Here's a note on the type of oil used: Grapeseed and canola are both mild-tasting oils high in monounsaturated fats. Olive oil would be too strong-tasting for this recipe. I don't ever recommend "vegetable oil," because that is a combination of various oils, most of them polyunsaturated (such as corn, soybean, or sunflower). Most people consume too many polyunsaturated oils and not enough mono-unsaturated, so choose olive, canola, and grapeseed when using oil. Even coconut oil is recommended over the polyunsaturated oils.

did you know?

Almonds are particularly high in vitamin E, which has been linked to reduced risk of heart disease, not only because of the antioxidant action of the vitamin but also because of the LDL lowering effect of almonds' monounsaturated fats. It's good fat, indeed.

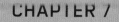

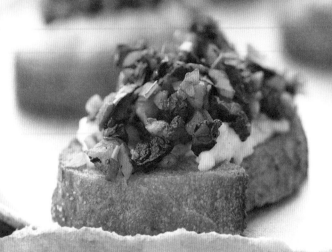

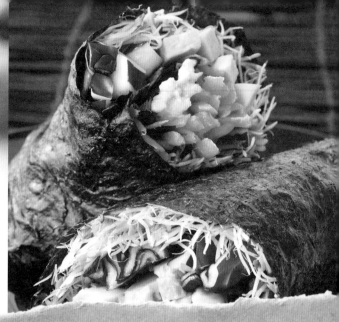

color me
BROWN/BLacK

COMFORT AND WARMTH MINGLED WITH DRAMA

When it comes to adding drama and contrast to a meal, black foods take the cake, and they're not too shabby from a nutritional standpoint either. Similarly, brown plant foods evoke warmth and comfort and abound in flavor, satisfying textures, and healthful properties.

Quite a few of the foods we're most familiar with have a black counterpart, including *black* sesame seeds, *black* rice, *black* radishes, and *black* carrots (see "Black Versions of Familiar Foods" on page 198 for a full list), but many black and brown foods are already in our repertoire: *black* beans, *brown* lentils, *black* olives, and *brown* … cocoa!

Rich in fiber, healthful fats, and antioxidants though they are, black and brown plant foods, especially mushrooms and sea vegetables, are absent from many people's diets. I'll grant that some people are averse to eating what are essentially fungi and algae, but the taste and health advantages supersede any squeamishness about their classifications.

As I emphasize over and over, the nutrients we need are *plant-based*, and this is especially true when it comes to minerals. Although most of us were indoctrinated to believe that minerals come from animal-based products, the opposite is true. By skipping the middleman (or rather, the middle *animal*), we can ensure intake and absorption of essential minerals, such as those abundant in the black and brown stars of this chapter.

Mushrooms

Rich in the mineral selenium, mushrooms play a significant role in reducing prostate cancer risk. According to the USDA, one serving of cremini (aka baby portobello) mushrooms provides almost one-third the Daily Value for selenium. Speaking of minerals, mushrooms are also an excellent source of potassium and copper. One medium portobello mushroom has even more potassium than a banana or a glass of orange juice, and one serving of mushrooms provides about 20 to 40 percent of the Daily Value of copper, a mineral that has cardioprotective properties.

Sea Vegetables

The thousands of types of sea vegetables come in brown, black, red, and green, each with a distinct shape, taste, and texture. In addition, they offer the broadest range of minerals of any food, especially iron, calcium, magnesium, and iodine. All too absent from our diets (and in our bodies) but readily available from the sea, these marine vegetables also contain such trace minerals as zinc, boron, selenium, and chromium. A few of the more familiar ones include the following:

• Nori is a dark purple/black sea vegetable that turns a phosphorescent green when heated and is most known for sushi rolls in Japanese cuisine.

• Kelp is light brown to dark green in color and often sold in flake form.

• Hijiki, a strikingly jet-black-colored sea vegetable, looks like small black wiry pasta.

- Kombu is very dark in color and generally sold in strips or sheets and is often used as a base for soup stocks.

- Wakame is similar to kombu and most commonly used to make miso soup.

- Arame is a lacy sea vegetable that is sweeter and milder in taste than many others and is good for the uninitiated.

- Dulse, which also tends to come in flake form, has a soft, chewy texture with a reddish brown color.

Chocolate

This antioxidant-rich plant-based food, appropriately placed in the brown chapter, is often lauded for its protective, healthful benefits, which pleases anyone with a chocolate addiction. So what's the scoop? Can chocolate be part of a healthful diet?

It's true that chocolate may benefit the heart in several ways. Cocoa (chocolate without the cocoa butter, which is where the fat naturally comes from) has an aspirin-like effect, helping to prevent blood clots and thus helping to prevent heart attacks. Cocoa also helps dilate blood vessels, which helps blood flow more easily, and a healthy cardiovascular system is really all about increased blood flow. More than that, the phytochemicals in cocoa, called flavonoids (also found in tea), are powerful antioxidants, thus reducing damage to coronary arteries.

Although cocoa butter (fat) is made up of a combination of monounsaturated fats as well as saturated fats, the latter do not raise blood cholesterol levels the way animal-based saturated fats do, and the former are responsible for lowering cholesterol levels. Moreover, some studies suggest that chocolate helps prevent the oxidation of LDL ("bad") cholesterol and its ensuing damage to coronary arteries.

Still, there has never been a study showing that chocolate actually prevents heart disease or other cardiovascular diseases. It's also important to keep in mind that much of the research around chocolate has been funded by the chocolate industry and tends to focus on cocoa or chocolate containing high levels of flavonoids, not the chocolate candy people tend to eat.

Commercial chocolates and cocoas are typically processed such that much of their phytochemicals are destroyed. They also often contain lots of sugar; and they also have added cow's milk in the case of "milk chocolate" and some dark chocolate (which, by definition, is not "dark chocolate"). In fact, there is evidence that any benefit derived from the phytochemicals is negated when cow's milk is added to chocolate or when cow's milk is consumed at the same time dark chocolate is consumed.

So, when choosing chocolate as part of a healthful diet, always go for a good-quality dark chocolate (the better brands should not include cow's milk or "milk powder") and keep in mind, particularly if you are trying to lose weight, that the calories in even the healthiest dark chocolate can add up. With that in mind, chocolate and cocoa can most certainly be enjoyed on a regular basis—without guilt. (I recommend choosing organic and Fair Trade when possible.)

advance preparation required

Arame and Cucumber Salad

▶ *Wheat-free*

Given to me by friend Alka Chandna many moons ago, this recipe stars arame,
a mild-tasting, black-colored sea vegetable.

½ cup (25 g) dried arame

2 tablespoons (30 ml) toasted sesame oil

1 to 2 teaspoons tamari soy sauce

2 tablespoons (30 ml) seasoned rice vinegar or
   1 tablespoon (15 ml) wine vinegar

1 tablespoon (15 ml) mirin

1½ cups (150 g) sliced radishes

1 cucumber, cut into matchsticks

½ cup (25 g) bean sprouts

1 tablespoon (8 g) toasted sesame seeds

DIRECTIONS

Soak the arame in a bowl of cold water for about
15 minutes or until rehydrated. Drain, rinse under
running water, and drain again. The arame will have
tripled in volume.

Place the arame in a saucepan with enough water
to immerse it. Bring to a boil and then reduce the
heat and simmer for about 30 minutes, or until
tender.

Meanwhile, combine the sesame oil, tamari, vinegar, and mirin in a small bowl and mix thoroughly.
Alternatively, you can add them to a small jar and
shake until thoroughly combined.

When the arame is finished cooking, drain to
remove any excess water. Add the arame, radishes,
cucumber, and bean sprouts to a bowl, drizzle with
the dressing, and toss gently.

Arrange on 4 small plates and serve.

YIELD: 4 servings

PER SERVING: 96 Calories; 8g Fat (64.9% calories from
fat); 2g Protein; 8g Carbohydrate; 2g Dietary Fiber; 0mg
Cholesterol; 147mg Sodium

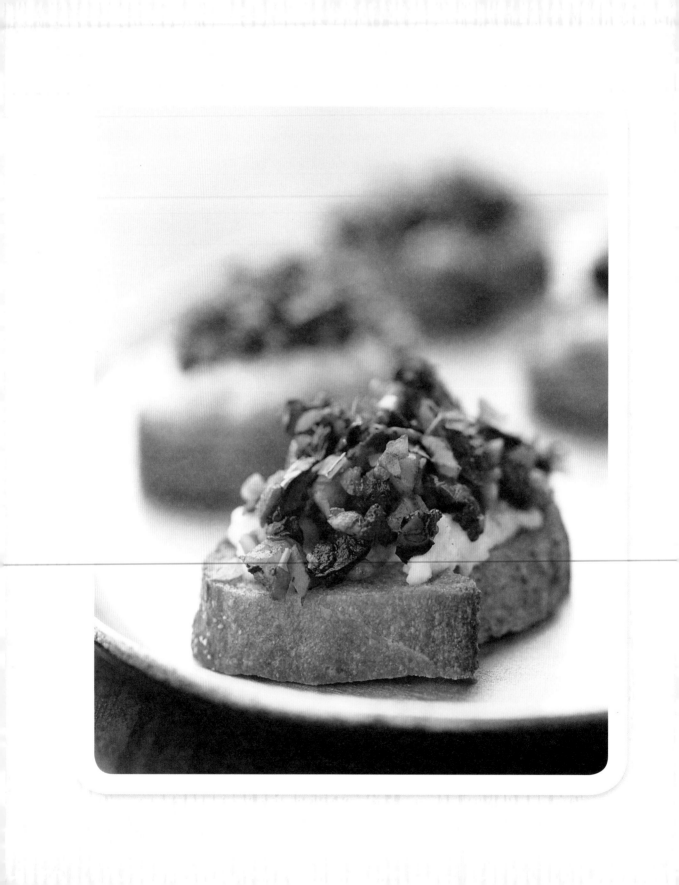

advance preparation required

Black Olive Bruschetta

▶ *Oil-free, wheat-free*

This is a beautiful and delicious appetizer. The contrast between the white cashew cream and black olives is striking—and even more so if you serve it along with traditional tomato bruschetta (see *The Vegan Table*, if you have it!).

BRUSCHETTA

2 tablespoons (30 ml) olive oil, plus more
   for brushing

3 cloves garlic, finely minced

2 shallots, finely minced

Salt and freshly ground pepper, to taste

¼ cup (35 g) pine nuts, coarsely chopped

½ cup (50 g) pitted black olives, finely minced

1 teaspoon balsamic vinegar

1 whole grain baguette, sliced

1 recipe Cashew Cream (see below)

1 tablespoon (4 g) finely minced fresh parsley

1 tablespoon (4 g) finely minced fresh basil

CASHEW CREAM

1 cup (150 g) raw cashews

1 tablespoon (15 ml) olive oil, plus more for
   brushing

½ yellow onion, finely chopped

1 teaspoon yellow/light miso

1 tablespoon (15 ml) lemon juice

1 tablespoon (15 ml) water

DIRECTIONS (CASHEW CREAM)

Soak the cashews overnight in enough water to cover them. The next day, drain and rinse the cashews. Set aside. In a medium sauté pan, heat the 1 tablespoon (15 ml) oil and sauté the onion until translucent and tender, 5 to 7 minutes.

Place the soaked cashews, sautéed onions, miso, lemon juice, and water into a blender and process until smooth.

DIRECTIONS (BRUSCHETTA)

Preheat the oven to 400°F (200°C, or gas mark 6). Line a baking sheet with unbleached parchment paper.

Add the 2 tablespoons (30 ml) oil to a large sauté pan, along with the garlic, shallots, and a pinch of salt and pepper. Cook over medium heat until the shallots begin to glisten, about 5 minutes. Stir in the pine nuts and olives and sauté for 3 minutes longer. Stir in the balsamic vinegar and turn off the heat.

Lightly brush both sides of the bread slices with oil. Arrange on the prepared baking sheet and bake until the ends of the bread begin to turn golden brown and crispy, 5 to 7 minutes.

Remove from the oven and let cool for 10 minutes. Spread a generous amount of cashew cream on each bread slice and carefully spoon the olive mixture on top. Sprinkle with some minced parsley and basil and arrange on a pretty serving platter.

YIELD: 20 servings, depending on size of baguette

PER SERVING: 119 Calories; 6g Fat (42.5% calories from fat); 3g Protein; 14g Carbohydrate; 1g Dietary Fiber; 0mg Cholesterol; 199mg Sodium

compassionate cooks' tip

You can make your olive mixture ahead of time and refrigerate it in an airtight container. You can also prepare your bread ahead and store in a separate airtight container. Assemble right before serving.

Olive Salad

▶ *Wheat-free, soy-free*

Olive lovers will relish this easy salad that is a perfect appetizer or meal starter.

¾ cup (170 g) pitted black olives, drained
¾ cup (170 g) pitted kalamata olives, drained
¾ cup (170 g) pitted green olives, drained
1 jar (6 ounces, or 170 g) marinated
   artichoke hearts
1 small red onion, finely chopped
3 scallions, finely chopped
3 cloves garlic, minced
1 tablespoon (9 g) capers, rinsed
¼ cup (60 ml) red wine vinegar
¼ cup (60 ml) olive oil
2 teaspoons finely chopped fresh or
   1 teaspoon dried oregano
2 teaspoons finely chopped fresh or
   1 teaspoon dried parsley
2 teaspoons finely chopped fresh or
   1 teaspoon dried basil
1 teaspoon crushed red pepper flakes
½ teaspoon freshly ground black pepper

DIRECTIONS

Place all the ingredients in a large bowl and toss to combine.

Place in the refrigerator to let the flavors marry for as little as 1 hour or as long as 1 week. Serve as an appetizer for a dinner party, as a side for a casual meal, or as a sandwich condiment or spread for crackers (see below).

YIELD: 12 servings, about ¼ cup (60 g) each

SERVING SUGGESTIONS AND VARIATIONS

To prepare as a condiment or spread, pulse the olives and artichoke hearts in a food processor before adding the rest of the ingredients and storing in the fridge. It will be much more "spreadable" and appropriate for a sandwich or crackers.

PER SERVING: 132 Calories; 12g Fat (80.2% calories from fat); 1g Protein; 6g Carbohydrate; 2g Dietary Fiber; 0mg Cholesterol; 536mg Sodium

compassionate cooks' tip

I prefer using fresh olives, choosing the best from the olive bar at my local grocery store. If you opt for canned olives, as a guide, ¾ cup is about how much is in the typical 5- or 6-ounce (140- or 170-g) can of olives.

Spicy Black Bean and Olive "Hummus"

▶ *Oil-free, wheat-free, soy-free*

Granted, the word *hummus* actually means "chickpea," but I decided against calling this a "dip" because many of the ingredients are those used in a traditional chickpea "hummus" recipe. On the other hand, it pairs better with tortilla chips than with pita bread or raw veggies. Try it, and you'll see what I mean.

1 can (15 ounces, or 420 g) black beans, drained and rinsed

10 black olives, pitted

1 small jalapeño pepper, finely chopped

1 or 2 cloves garlic, peeled and left whole, divided

2 tablespoons (30 ml) lemon juice, divided

1½ tablespoons (24 g) sesame tahini

½ teaspoon ground cumin

½ teaspoon salt

¼ teaspoon cayenne pepper

Paprika or chili powder, for garnish

DIRECTIONS

Add the beans, olives, pepper, 1 of the garlic cloves, 1 tablespoon (15 ml) of the lemon juice, tahini, cumin, salt, and cayenne pepper to a food processor or blender. Process or blend until smooth, scraping down the sides as needed. Taste and adjust the seasonings as necessary, adding the remaining garlic clove and 1 tablespoon (15 ml) lemon juice, if desired. Garnish with paprika and serve.

YIELD: 1¼ cups (280 g)

SERVING SUGGESTIONS AND VARIATIONS

- Use black tahini, which is made with black sesame seeds.
- Omit the jalapeño if you don't like spicy food.

PER SERVING: 58 Calories; 2g Fat (32.8% calories from fat); 3g Protein; 7g Carbohydrate; 3g Dietary Fiber; 0mg Cholesterol; 280mg Sodium

did you know?

There are natural and artificial methods of curing ripe and unripe olives. Ripe olives are either fermented in brine/salt water (Greek method), rubbed with coarse salt, and left to cure (resulting in a wrinkled appearance), or sun-cured (leaving fully ripe black olives on the tree to dry). Unripe green olives are soaked in a fast-acting lye solution for 6 to 16 hours (Spanish method) or soaked in an alkaline lye solution with iron added to preserve the dark color (American method).

Canned black olives are made from unripe olives, which are picked green, cured in lye, and pumped with oxygen to make them black.

BLACK VERSIONS OF FAMILIAR FOODS

Determined to highlight foods that are familiar to people, I made a point to not include recipes full of plant foods that are novel just because of their color. Although such foods as purple potatoes and blue cornmeal may require a little effort to find, I didn't want that to be the case for too many of the recipes. I figured if it would be difficult for *me* to find in the foodie-oriented, farmers'-market-rich, agriculture-heavy San Francisco Bay Area, then it would be difficult for people living elsewhere.

However, it would be a lost opportunity if I didn't at least mention some plant foods that have a dark side to their more traditionally known colors. That is to say, though we associate carrots with the color orange, rice with the color brown (hopefully, not white!), and sesame seeds with the color tan, each of these plant foods—and many others—have black counterparts. Look for them at a specialty store near you or online.

Black carrots: As you'll learn when you read about carrots on page 57, carrots were not originally orange. They were white, yellow, or purple, almost black, and these cultivars are making their way back into the marketplace (and my garden) these days.

Black walnuts: This variety has a rich, robust, almost smoky flavor. Although the husks are black, the nut meat is the same as that of the more familiar English walnut.

Black vinegar: Unlike balsamic vinegar, which is made from grapes, black vinegars begin with grains, typically sorghum, millet, wheat, and rice.

Black sesame seeds: The color of sesame seeds range from a creamy white to a charcoal black, and it's the latter I often use to add contrast to a brightly colored dish.

Black rice (a.k.a. Forbidden Rice): The deep black color in this gorgeous iron-rich rice is from—you guessed it—anthocyanins.

Black quinoa (KEEN-wa): Just when I thought I couldn't love this ancient grain more, I discovered its black counterpart. It's beautiful and nutritious.

Black dates: A staple food in the Middle East, dates have a number of different cultivars, including the black Hayany (from Egypt) and the black Dayri (from Iraq).

Black soybeans: This variety of the typically yellow soybean is perfect when any type of bean is called for in a recipe, especially black beans.

Black radishes: More widely eaten in Eastern Europe than in the United States, these pungent radishes have black peels but white flesh and can be cooked like turnips or eaten raw.

Black mushrooms and fungi: Although edible mushrooms and fungi come in a variety of white, tan, and brown hues, some are strikingly black, including black chanterelle, black Chinese mushrooms, and cloud ears.

Mushroom Barley Soup

▶ *Soy-free, wheat-free, and oil-free if sautéing in water and not using truffle oil*

Without a doubt, this is one of my absolute favorite soups. Perfect for a chilly, rainy night, it's a hearty soup with a robust flavor, particularly from the addition of the truffle oil.

4 cups (940 ml) water

¾ cup (150 g) uncooked pearl barley

2 medium onions, chopped

2 stalks celery, chopped

1 tablespoon (15 ml) oil or water, for sautéing

1½ pounds (683 g) sliced fresh mushrooms (shiitake and cremini are my favorites)

2 cups (260 g) chopped carrots (3 or 4 large carrots)

6 cups (1410 ml) mushroom or vegetable stock (or half of each)

1 tablespoon (15 g) tomato paste

1 tablespoon (15 ml) truffle oil

½ teaspoon salt

¼ teaspoon freshly ground pepper

3 tablespoons (12 g) minced fresh parsley

DIRECTIONS

In a 3-quart (3 L) saucepan, bring the water and barley to a boil. Reduce the heat; cover and simmer for 30 minutes or until the barley is partially cooked. Drain.

Meanwhile, in a soup pot, sauté the onions and celery in oil until tender, about 7 minutes. Add the mushrooms; cook, stirring, for 5 to 10 minutes. Stir in the carrots, stock, tomato paste, and partially cooked barley.

Bring to a boil over medium heat. Reduce the heat; cover and simmer for 30 minutes, stirring occasionally. Stir in truffle oil, salt, and pepper. Taste and adjust the seasonings.

Sprinkle with parsley and serve.

YIELD: 6 servings

PER SERVING: 194 Calories; 4g Fat (19.0% calories from fat); 6g Protein; 36g Carbohydrate; 7g Dietary Fiber; 0mg Cholesterol; 1230mg Sodium

compassionate cooks' tip

Because they'll get soggy very quickly, mushrooms should never be washed and then put in a bag until ready to use. A little wipe with a moist towel is enough to remove any lingering soil, or if you're going to use them right away, rinsing them with water is just fine.

did you know?

Shiitake mushrooms (as well as oyster, king oyster, and maitake) have been found to be a top source of potent antioxidants, particularly one called L-ergothioneine. Providing cellular protection, this antioxidant is also found in portobellos and creminis, followed by white buttons.

Five-Spice Onion Soup

▶ *Wheat-free*

This is a surprisingly hearty soup for one that is not creamy or puréed. The broth is much healthier than that of a traditional French onion soup (which this one reminds me of), thanks to all the yummy spices. Don't be intimidated by the number of ingredients. It's a very simple soup to prepare.

1 tablespoon (15 ml) water or oil, for sautéing

1 yellow onion, coarsely chopped

6 cups (1410 ml) vegetable stock

½ inch (1.3 cm) fresh ginger, peeled and sliced

6 whole cloves

1 cinnamon stick

½ teaspoon aniseed

½ teaspoon fennel seeds

1 tablespoon (15 ml) tamari soy sauce

1 tablespoon (20 g) molasses

2 tablespoons (28 g) nondairy butter (such as Earth Balance)

2 large yellow onions, thinly sliced

1 tablespoon (13 g) granulated sugar

6 cloves garlic, minced

Salt and freshly ground pepper, to taste

DIRECTIONS

Heat the water in a soup pot and add the chopped onion. Sauté over medium heat for 5 minutes, stirring frequently, until translucent.

Add the vegetable stock, ginger, cloves, cinnamon stick, aniseed, fennel seeds, tamari, and molasses. Stir to combine. Bring to a boil, reduce the heat to medium-low, and simmer for 20 minutes, uncovered.

Meanwhile, in a large sauté pan, melt the nondairy butter over medium heat. Add the 2 sliced onions and sugar and cook until the onions begin to brown, stirring occasionally. Depending on the pan you're using and the heat of your stove, this could take 15 to 30 minutes. The onions should be golden brown and caramelized before adding them to the soup. When the onions are almost done, add the garlic, and continue to sauté until the garlic is golden brown. Remove from the heat.

Strain out and discard all the solid ingredients from the broth and return the broth to the soup pot. Add the caramelized onions and garlic to the broth, season with salt and pepper to taste, and simmer over low heat until ready to serve.

YIELD: 6 to 8 servings

SERVING SUGGESTIONS AND VARIATIONS

• Favorite additions to this soup include 6 medium shiitake mushrooms, sliced; extra-firm tofu, cubed; or a dash of truffle oil, added at the very end.

• Star anise is a fine substitute if you have trouble finding aniseed.

Hot and Sour Soup

▶ *Wheat-free*

One of my husband's favorite soups in Chinese restaurants, this delicious version features a couple different types of black and brown mushrooms, though any variety will do.

1 ounce (28 g) dried wood ear or cloud
   ear mushrooms

6 dried shiitake mushrooms

2 cups (470 ml) hot water

4 cups (940 ml) vegetable stock

¼ teaspoon crushed red pepper flakes

1 teaspoon freshly ground black pepper

3 tablespoons (45 ml) tamari soy sauce

¼ cup (60 ml) rice vinegar, seasoned or regular

¼ cup (32 g) cornstarch

12 ounces (340 g) firm or extra-firm tofu,
   cubed or cut into strips

½ cup (60 g) bamboo shoots, cut into strips

2 teaspoons chili oil

2 teaspoons sesame oil

3 scallions, finely chopped

did you know?

Mushrooms contain an abundance of selenium, a trace mineral linked with cancer prevention, and they are an excellent source of potassium, riboflavin, and niacin.

DIRECTIONS

Place the wood ear and shiitake mushrooms in a medium bowl along with the hot water. Soak for 20 minutes until they are rehydrated. Drain but reserve the liquid. Cut away the mushroom stems and slice the caps into thin strips.

In a large saucepan or soup pot, add the reserved mushroom liquid along with the vegetable stock and bring to a boil over medium heat. Stir in the sliced mushrooms. Reduce the heat to a simmer, and cook for 5 minutes. Stir in the red pepper flakes and black pepper.

Meanwhile, in a medium bowl, combine the tamari, rice vinegar, and cornstarch and whisk until the cornstarch is completely dissolved. Add it to the soup pot and stir until the mixture begins to thicken, 3 to 5 minutes.

Increase the heat to a medium-low boil and add the tofu, bamboo shoots, chili oil, and sesame oil. Cook for about 5 minutes to heat the tofu through and serve hot in individual bowls, topped with the scallions.

YIELD: 4 servings

PER SERVING: 188 Calories; 9g Fat (40.5% calories from fat); 9g Protein; 21g Carbohydrate; 3g Dietary Fiber; 0mg Cholesterol; 1194mg Sodium

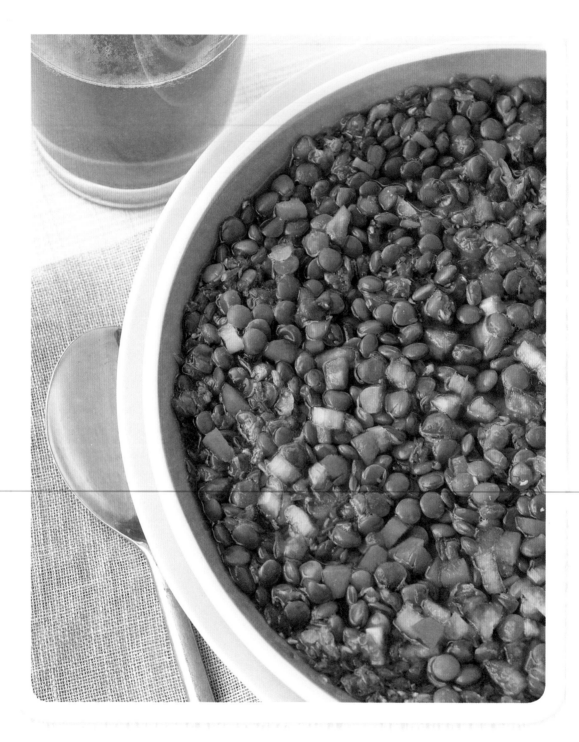

Brown Lentil Soup

▶ *Oil-free if sautéing in water and omitting the truffle oil, soy-free, wheat-free*

Being semi-puréed, this soup is both smooth and textured. It's hearty, nutritious, and full of flavor.

2 tablespoons (30 ml) water or oil, for sautéing

1 large yellow onion, chopped

3 cloves garlic, finely chopped

2 carrots, finely chopped

2 stalks celery, finely chopped

2 cups (400 g) brown lentils, picked through and rinsed

8 cups (1880 ml) vegetable stock

1 teaspoon salt, plus more to taste

½ teaspoon freshly ground coriander

½ teaspoon freshly ground cumin

2 tomatoes, seeded and chopped

1 tablespoon (15 ml) truffle oil (optional)

Freshly ground pepper, to taste

Chopped fresh parsley, for garnish

DIRECTIONS

Heat the water in a soup pot over medium heat. Add the onion, garlic, carrots, and celery and cook until the onion is translucent, about 7 minutes.

Add the lentils, stock, 1 teaspoon salt, coriander, and cumin and stir to combine. Increase the heat to high and bring to a boil. Reduce the heat to medium-low, cover, and cook until the lentils are tender, 35 to 40 minutes.

Using an immersion blender, purée to your preferred consistency. Alternatively, you may transfer a portion of the soup to the blender, purée, and then return to the pot.

Add the tomatoes to the semi-puréed soup and stir to combine. Add the truffle oil, taste for seasonings, and add more salt if necessary.

Serve hot topped with freshly ground pepper and chopped parsley.

YIELD: 6 to 8 servings

PER SERVING: 244 Calories; 5g Fat (18.7% calories from fat); 15g Protein; 37g Carbohydrate; 17g Dietary Fiber; 0mg Cholesterol; 1283mg Sodium

compassionate cooks' tip

To avoid a bitter flavor, never purchase onions that have begun to sprout greens from their stem side. This indicates they are old and no longer fresh.

Black Beluga Lentil Salad

▶ *Wheat-free, soy-free*

Called such because they resemble the eggs of the beluga whale when cooked, these nutritious pulses do have a striking appearance in their shiny blackness.

1 cup (200 g) dried black beluga or
  French Puy lentils
2½ cups (588 ml) vegetable stock
2 carrots, finely chopped
3 scallions, chopped
1 tablespoon (4 g) chopped fresh parsley
1 tablespoon (4 g) chopped fresh oregano
  or (6 g) marjoram
½ cup (75 g) chopped toasted almonds
2 tablespoons (30 ml) olive oil
3 tablespoons (45 ml) good-quality
  balsamic vinegar
½ teaspoon salt, or to taste
Freshly ground pepper, to taste

DIRECTIONS

Rinse the lentils in a strainer and pick through to remove any stones or debris.

Add the lentils and stock to a 3-quart (3 L) saucepan, and turn the heat to medium-low. Cover, and simmer for 30 minutes until the lentils are tender. Check halfway through the cooking time to make sure the stock hasn't evaporated. If you need to, add additional water to prevent the lentils from burning. Remove from the heat, drain any excess water (reserving the stock for another use), and transfer to a large mixing bowl.

You can wait for the lentils to cool, but I don't bother because I like to serve it warm. To the lentils, add the carrots, scallions, parsley, oregano, almonds, olive oil, balsamic vinegar, salt, and pepper. Stir to combine and taste.

Add any more seasonings, as needed, and either serve right away or store in the refrigerator for a few hours or overnight. You may need to refresh it with additional vinegar or salt before serving. Also, I prefer to bring it to room temperature before serving.

Serve as a side or starter or atop a bed of spinach or mixed greens.

YIELD: 4 servings

SERVING SUGGESTIONS AND VARIATIONS

- As mentioned in the ingredients, French Puy lentils can be used instead of beluga lentils. These are the two lentils I'd recommend for this dish because they both hold their shape after being cooked, but small black beans also work well.
- You may use sliced or julienned almonds instead of chopped.

PER SERVING: 358 Calories; 18g Fat (42.8% calories from fat); 16g Protein; 37g Carbohydrate; 4g Dietary Fiber; 0mg Cholesterol; 905mg Sodium

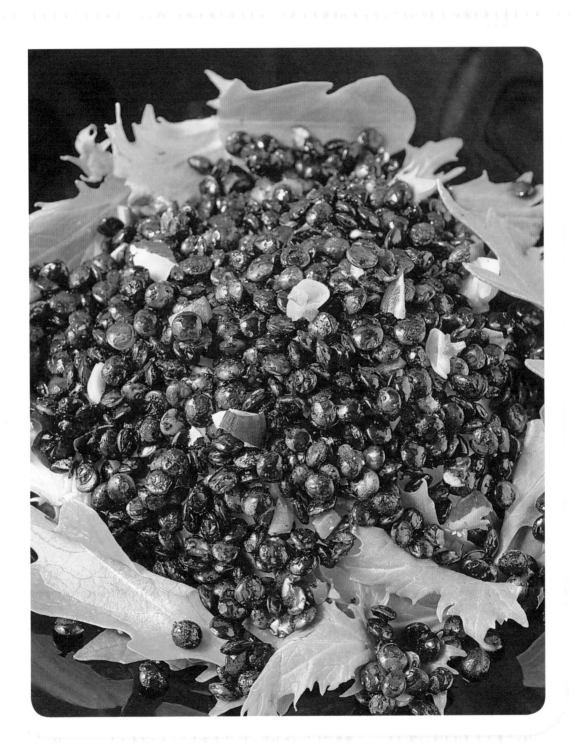

Shiitake Mushroom Gravy

A bit of an Asian variation on my simple gravy recipe (see Golden Gravy in *The Vegan Table*), this one pairs equally well with mashed potatoes, bread stuffing, or anything else you'd like to add it to.

3 tablespoon (45 ml) sesame oil, divided
1 yellow onion, sliced
1 tablespoon (10 g) minced garlic
1 cup (70 g) thinly sliced shiitake mushrooms
2 tablespoons (16 g) flour
2 tablespoons (30 ml) water
2 cups (470 ml) vegetable stock
2 tablespoons (30 ml) tamari soy sauce,
   or to taste

compassionate cooks' tip

Admittedly, I was a mushroom hater for much of my adult life, but it was the shiitake mushroom that made me see the light. If you try just one mushroom, try the shiitake. It is incredibly flavorful with a wonderful chewy texture. Sautéed in a little sesame oil, shiitake mushrooms make a wonderful addition to soups, salads, and stir-fries.

DIRECTIONS

Heat 1 tablespoon (15 ml) of the sesame oil in a large sauté pan over medium-high heat. Add the onion and garlic and cook until the onion begins to turn translucent, about 5 minutes, stirring occasionally.

Add the mushrooms and cook for 10 more minutes, stirring occasionally, until the mushrooms are cooked.

Meanwhile, add the flour, remaining 2 tablespoons (30 ml) oil, and water to a small bowl and whisk until a thick paste is formed. Set aside.

Add the vegetable stock and tamari to the cooking mushrooms and stir to combine. Add the flour/water combination and cook for 10 minutes over low heat until the gravy develops a thick consistency.

YIELD: 20 servings, about 2 tablespoons (30 ml) each

SERVING SUGGESTIONS AND VARIATIONS
Purée all or half of the finished gravy.

PER SERVING: 34 Calories; 2g Fat (54.9% calories from fat); trace Protein; 4g Carbohydrate; trace Dietary Fiber; 0mg Cholesterol; 125mg Sodium

Onion Gravy

▶ *Wheat-free, soy-free and oil-free if using soy-free Earth Balance*

The richest-tasting gravy comes from slowly browned onions. This is a simple recipe that can be doubled as easily as it can be tripled.

2 tablespoons (28 g) nondairy butter
  (such as Earth Balance) or oil
2 large yellow onions, diced or sliced
½ teaspoon salt
1 cup (235 ml) vegetable stock

compassionate cooks' tip

Here are some helpful conversions that might aid you in your kitchen:

1 small onion = 1 tablespoon dried minced onions or ½ tablespoon onion powder

1 pound (455 g) onions = 4 medium onions or 4 cups chopped/sliced onions

1 medium onion = 1 cup (160 g) chopped/sliced onion

DIRECTIONS

In a large sauté pan, heat the butter over medium heat. Add the onions and cook until they begin to brown, stirring occasionally. Keep the pan uncovered; otherwise, you will add moisture, which will slow down the caramelizing process.

Continue cooking until the onions begin to brown, reducing the heat to medium-low. Depending on the size of your onions and the strength of your heat, the process could take anywhere from 15 to 30 minutes. Be sure to stir occasionally.

Once they are as brown as you like them (it's really up to you), add the salt and turn the heat to low, if you haven't already. Stir.

Pour the vegetable stock into the pan and stir to combine. Bring the mixture to a simmer and continue to simmer for 10 minutes, stirring occasionally; as the stock begins to evaporate the mixture thickens. If it is not as thick as you like it after 10 minutes, give it another 10 minutes.

Serve hot over mashed potatoes, baked potatoes, grilled tempeh, baked tofu, or grilled mushrooms.

YIELD: 8 servings, about 2 tablespoons (30 ml) each

SERVING SUGGESTIONS AND VARIATIONS
- Use half broth and half red or white wine.
- Add some fresh or dried herbs when you add the stock for some extra flavor.

PER SERVING: 37 Calories; 3g Fat (67.1% calories from fat); trace Protein; 3g Carbohydrate; trace Dietary Fiber; 0mg Cholesterol; 258mg Sodium

Mushroom-Topped Baked Potatoes

▶ *Wheat-free, soy-free if using soy-free Earth Balance*

A simple meal when you want optimum nutrition but familiar comfort food, this is definitely a mushroom-lover's dish.

2 large baking potatoes

Oil, for coating potatoes

Salt and freshly ground pepper, to taste

1 tablespoon (14 g) nondairy butter (such as Earth Balance) or oil

8 ounces (225 g) fresh mushrooms (cremini, shiitake, or any favorite), sliced

1 red bell pepper, seeded and cut into 1-inch (2.5 cm) squares

1 large clove garlic, minced

¼ cup (60 ml) water or vegetable stock

1 tablespoon (15 ml) lemon juice

Chopped fresh parsley, for garnish

DIRECTIONS

Preheat the oven to 350°F (180°C, or gas mark 4).

Rub the potato skins with a bit of olive oil and salt. (This yields a crispy skin when they're done baking.) Poke some fork holes into the raw potatoes, place on the center rack of your oven, and bake until the potatoes are crispy on the outside and soft on the inside, about 1 hour.

Heat the butter in a large sauté pan over medium-high heat. Add the mushrooms, bell pepper, and garlic. Toss until the mushrooms brown lightly. Add the water and lemon juice and reduce the heat to low. Cook and stir for about 3 minutes. Season with salt and pepper.

Split and fluff the potatoes. Top with the hot mushroom mixture. Sprinkle with the chopped parsley, and serve.

YIELD: 2 servings

SERVING SUGGESTION AND VARIATION

To make the mushrooms a little creamier, add ¼ cup (60 ml) vegetable stock to the mushrooms as they cook.

PER SERVING: 245 Calories; 6g Fat (21.1% calories from fat); 7g Protein; 44g Carbohydrate; 5g Dietary Fiber; 0mg Cholesterol; 144mg Sodium

Drunken Beans
(*Frijoles Borrachos*)

▶ *Wheat-free, soy-free, oil-free if sautéing in water*

An excellent source of protein, iron, potassium, fiber, and folate, pinto beans take center stage in this hearty dish. This is comfort food at its best—Mexican style.

1 tablespoon (15 ml) oil or water, for sautéing

1 yellow onion, diced

1 green bell pepper, seeded and diced

4 jalapeño or serrano peppers, seeded and diced

3 cloves garlic, minced

1½ teaspoons ground cumin

3 tablespoons (23 g) chili powder

6 cups (1,026 g) cooked pinto beans or 4 cans (14 ounces, or 395 g), drained and rinsed

1 bottle (8 ounces, or 235 ml) Dos Equis or other Mexican beer

3 tablespoons (45 g) light or dark brown sugar

1 teaspoon salt, or to taste

8 grinds black pepper

⅓ cup (5 g) chopped fresh cilantro or (20 g) parsley

DIRECTIONS

Heat the oil in a large pot. Add the onion and sauté until soft, about 5 minutes. Add the bell pepper, jalapeño peppers, garlic, cumin, and chili powder and cook for 5 minutes longer, stirring occasionally.

Add the beans, beer, brown sugar, salt, and pepper and simmer for 20 to 30 minutes. At the end of the cooking time, stir in the cilantro and remove from the heat. Serve hot.

YIELD: 8 servings

SERVING SUGGESTIONS AND VARIATIONS

Serve with tortilla chips, salsa, and cubed avocado or nondairy sour cream.

PER SERVING: 228 Calories; 3g Fat (11.9% calories from fat); 10g Protein; 40g Carbohydrate; 9g Dietary Fiber; 0mg Cholesterol; 1128mg Sodium

food lore

Most people have seen cooked pinto beans, which boast a pink color, but before they're cooked, the reason for their name is more obvious: their beige background is strewn with reddish brown splashes of color making them look "painted," which is what *pinto* means in Spanish.

did you know?

One cup of cooked pinto beans provides almost 60 percent of the recommended daily intake for fiber. Research studies have shown that insoluble fiber not only helps increase stool bulk and prevent constipation but also helps prevent digestive disorders such as irritable bowel syndrome, diverticulosis, and diverticulitis.

Peanut Butter Pancakes

▶ *Soy-free and oil-free if using soy-free milk and Earth Balance*

Perhaps it's just an excuse to eat one of my favorite foods, but the peanut butter does add nice flavor, healthful fat, and healthful plant protein. Plus, kids love it!

1¼ cups (150 g) all-purpose flour

2 tablespoons (25 g) granulated sugar

1 tablespoon (14 g) baking powder

½ teaspoon salt

1¼ cups (295 ml) nondairy milk (such as almond, soy, rice, hazelnut, hemp, or oat)

¼ cup (65 g) natural peanut butter

2 tablespoons (30 ml) oil or (28 g) nondairy butter (such as Earth Balance)

DIRECTIONS

In a medium bowl, combine the flour, sugar, baking powder, and salt.

In a small bowl or measuring cup, stir together the milk and peanut butter until smooth. Add to the dry ingredients and beat just until a batter is formed. Do not overbeat.

Lightly oil a nonstick sauté pan or griddle over medium heat. Spoon the batter by ¼ cupfuls into the pan. Cook until golden brown on both sides. Serve immediately.

YIELD: 8 to 10 servings

SERVING SUGGESTIONS AND VARIATIONS

- Other nut butters work just as well; just make sure they're nice and smooth before adding.
- Testers insisted I suggest adding a handful of non-dairy chocolate chips to the batter, as well as ripe banana slices.

PER SERVING: 142 Calories; 7g Fat (43.2% calories from fat); 4g Protein; 16g Carbohydrate; 1g Dietary Fiber; 0mg Cholesterol; 220mg Sodium

Almond Butter and Strawberry Sandwich

▶ *Oil-free, soy-free, wheat-free if using wheat-free bread*

Here's a quick idea for incorporating red (strawberries), yellow (bananas), and brown (fiber-rich bread and almond butter) foods into an all-in-one, portable meal.

3 tablespoons (48 g) natural almond butter
2 slices whole-grain bread
2 fresh strawberries, sliced
½ banana, peeled and sliced
2 tablespoons (40 g) strawberry jam or
    preserves, sweetened naturally

DIRECTIONS

Spread the almond butter over one side of one slice of bread. Arrange the strawberries and bananas on top of the almond butter.

Spread the jam on one side of the remaining slice of bread. Place over the fruit to make a sandwich.

YIELD: 1 sandwich

SERVING SUGGESTIONS AND VARIATIONS

- Use cashew, hazelnut, macadamia, soy nut, peanut, hemp seed, or sunflower seed butter.
- Sprinkle a little ground cinnamon on the bananas.
- Instead of bananas, add other sliced fruit, such as apples, figs, or pears.

PER SERVING: 669 Calories; 32g Fat (40.6% calories from fat); 16g Protein; 90g Carbohydrate; 10g Dietary Fiber; 0mg Cholesterol; 465mg Sodium

compassionate cooks' tips

- Make this a day ahead, wrap well in plastic, and refrigerate.

- I always urge people to choose nut and seed butters without added oil and sugar. A little salt is okay, but the ingredients should say nothing more than "roasted almonds, salt" or "raw hazelnuts, salt," for example. Although the natural oils tend to separate from the seeds or nuts, they are easy to stir and use. To avoid oil spillage over the top of the jar, simply turn the covered jar upside down for a few hours so the oil migrates to the bottom. Then flip the jar back over, open, and stir.

Nori Wraps with Orange Cashew Cream

▶ *Oil-free, wheat-free*

Light but filling, flavorful but simple, these wraps are my favorite summertime dish. The color of the nori sheets is a dark, shiny, green—almost black—and adds a striking contrast to the colorful filling.

ORANGE CASHEW CREAM

1 cup (150 g) raw cashews

½ to ¾ cup (120 to 175 ml) fresh squeezed orange juice

1 to 2 tablespoons (15 to 30 ml) tamari soy sauce

WRAPS

4 nori sheets (the kind used for sushi; found in the Asian section of a grocery store)

2 carrots, grated or shredded

1 medium beet, grated

¼ head red or green cabbage, shredded

¼ cup (12 g) alfalfa sprouts

2 avocados, sliced or mashed

Salt, for sprinkling

Black sesame seeds, for garnish

DIRECTIONS

To make the cashew cream, add the cashews, ½ cup (120 ml) of the orange juice, and tamari to a blender and blend until you have a creamy consistency. Taste, tweak if necessary, thin out with more juice, if needed, and then transfer to a bowl.

To make the wraps, set out all your grated veggies in separate bowls so you can grab them as needed to make your wraps.

Place a nori sheet on the counter or cutting board. Leaving a 1-inch (2.5 cm) border at each edge of the nori sheet, place a thin layer of grated carrot, grated beet, shredded cabbage, and alfalfa sprouts on top of the nori sheet. Place the avocado in a horizontal line across the middle of the shredded veggies and do the same with the cashew sauce. Sprinkle on a little salt.

Working from the bottom, roll up the nori like a fat cigar, tucking in the veggies as you roll upward. You should have a neatly packed cylinder at the end. Use a little water to "seal" the seam. Serve as a wrap or use a sharp serrated knife to cut into 1½-inch (3.8 cm) rounds. Repeat with the remaining ingredients. You should have enough veggies to make 4 wraps. Sprinkle with black sesame seeds for a pretty presentation.

YIELD: 4 wraps and ¾ cup (270 g) dressing

SERVING SUGGESTIONS AND VARIATIONS
If you do not like nori, use large lettuce leaves or whole raw or steamed collard leaves.

PER SERVING: 352 Calories; 26g Fat (62.7% calories from fat); 8g Protein; 26g Carbohydrate; 6g Dietary Fiber; 0mg Cholesterol; 309mg Sodium

compassionate cooks' tip

Because the nori gets soft when it is wet, it is best to serve the wraps as soon as they are prepared.

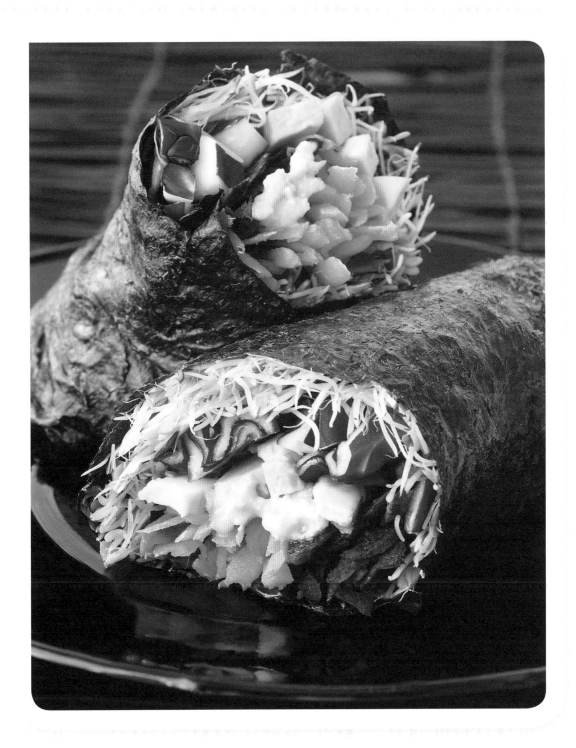

advance preparation required

Double Chocolate Mint Granita

▶ *Soy-free, wheat-free, oil-free*

Since I already included sorbets and shakes in my previous cookbooks, I thought I'd include granitas in this one. They're lighter, icier versions of sorbet that are less fussy to make. Although you will find a fruit-based version in the Watermelon Granita (page 38), this chocolate version is a little more decadent.

4 cups (940 ml) water
⅔ cup (132 g) granulated sugar
1 cup (120 g) unsweetened cocoa
¼ cup (45 g) nondairy semisweet
   chocolate chips
¼ teaspoon peppermint extract
Fresh mint sprigs or leaves, for garnish

did you know?

Much has been made of chocolate's healthful properties, particularly as they relate to chocolate's flavonoids, the same group of phytochemicals found in tea and red wine. And though it's true that all plants have beneficial properties, most of the research uses cocoa or chocolate containing higher levels of flavonoids than you'll ever eat in a typical chocolate bar. Besides, most chocolate is processed in ways that destroy much of their phytochemicals; they also often contain milk fat (in milk chocolate), which negates the healthful properties, and lots of sugar. White chocolate contains no flavonoids at all.

DIRECTIONS

Add the water to a medium saucepan over medium-low heat and whisk in the sugar and cocoa. Cook, whisking, until the sugar and cocoa are thoroughly combined and the mixture starts to bubble a bit, 10 to 15 minutes.

Add the chocolate chips and stir until melted. Remove from the heat and add the peppermint extract. Stir to combine. Cool for about 15 minutes. (The cooler it is when you put it in the freezer, the faster it will freeze.)

Pour the chocolate mixture into a shallow, wide container and freeze for 1 hour. Rake the mixture with a fork and freeze for another hour. Rake and freeze for 1 more hour. The liquid should be frozen by this point. The entire process takes about 3 hours.

When ready to serve, rake it one more time to loosen the granita and spoon it into pretty glass bowls, margarita glasses, or wine goblets. Garnish with the mint sprigs. This may be held in the freezer for up to 2 days.

YIELD: 6 servings

PER SERVING: 198 Calories; 4g Fat (18.0% calories from fat); 5g Protein; 37g Carbohydrate; 6g Dietary Fiber; 0mg Cholesterol; 16mg Sodium

Chocolate Zucchini Bread

▶ *Soy-free*

My good friend Robin Brande, author of *Fat Cat*, sent me this delicious recipe, originally given to her by Michigan librarian Elizabeth Norton, who veganized her recipe just for Robin, who was accepting an award from the Michigan Library Association. Nothing like passing along a good thing!

3 tablespoons (21 g) ground flaxseed (equivalent of 3 eggs)

9 tablespoons (135 ml) water

3 cups (360 g) all-purpose or whole wheat pastry flour

¼ cup (30 g) unsweetened cocoa powder

1 tablespoon (8 g) ground cinnamon

1 teaspoon baking soda

½ teaspoon baking powder

1 teaspoon salt

2 cups (400 g) granulated sugar

1 cup (235 ml) canola oil

1 teaspoon pure vanilla extract

2 cups ((240 g) shredded zucchini (2 to 3 medium zucchini)

1 cup (150 g) chopped walnuts or other favorite nut (optional)

12 ounces (340 g) nondairy semi-sweet or dark chocolate chips

DIRECTIONS

Preheat the oven to 350°F (180°C, or gas mark 4). Lightly grease two 9 x 5-inch (23 x 13 cm) loaf pans with oil.

In a food processor or in a bowl using an electric hand mixer, whip the flaxseed and water together until you have a thick and creamy consistency. This can all be done by hand, but a food processor or hand mixer does a better job in about 1 to 2 minutes. It also makes it creamier than can be done by hand.

In a large bowl, combine the flour, cocoa, cinnamon, baking soda, baking powder, and salt. Mix well.

In a separate bowl, mix the flax eggs and the sugar until well combined. Add the oil and vanilla. Beat to combine and then stir in the zucchini.

Add the wet ingredients to the dry and stir until just combined. Fold in the nuts and chocolate chips.

Spoon into the loaf pans, dividing evenly between them. Bake for 55 to 60 minutes or until a toothpick inserted into the center comes out clean. Cool for 30 to 40 minutes in the pan then turn out onto racks.

YIELD: 2 loaves

PER SERVING: 318 Calories; 18g Fat (48.1% calories from fat); 5g Protein; 79g Carbohydrate; 3g Dietary Fiber; 0mg Cholesterol; 158mg Sodium

compassionate cooks' tips

- You might want to remove the seeds of the zucchini, especially from larger ones where the seeds might be bitter.

- This bread freezes very well.

- Use less sugar if that's your preference.

THE MANY COLORS OF TEA

When I was young, I drank a lot of black tea, a lot of generic, bagged black tea, fortifying it with a ton of sugar. That was many moons ago, and I'm glad to say I've gotten away from that habit. Today, I drink mostly green, white, and sometimes oolong. The only black tea I drink is technically "red," from my favorite tea house, Teance.

Evidence about tea's healthful properties is strong. Because the first people to study the relationship between tea and health were the Chinese and Japanese, they focused on the type of tea they drink: green. Green tea indeed deserves its lofty reputation, but evidence is mounting that black and other color teas are just as healthful.

The thing to know about the different types of tea is that they all come from the same plant, the *Camellia sinensis*, an evergreen shrub or small tree indigenous to China but also grown in other parts of the world, including South America, Indonesia, New Zealand, and Australia.

The difference in the teas just has to do with what they do to the leaves.

White tea: White tea represents the most natural form of teas processed for consumption. Steamed instead of air-dried to stop the oxidation process (which naturally begins occurring once the leaves are picked), white teas are plucked from the downy premature leaves of the white tea varietal and also include some buds. Picked just before the buds have opened, the tea takes its name from the silver fuzz that still covers the buds. Based on Western medical findings, white teas are reputed to be higher in antioxidants than green teas, and they're extremely low in caffeine.

Green tea: The next grade is green tea. Green teas have been pan-fired or steamed to retain their color and nutrients, and indeed, green teas have been found to be rich in antioxidants, vitamins, and nutrients. Reputed to increase concentration and prevent heart disease, osteoporosis, and many types of cancer, green tea can taste sweet, nutty, buttery, smoky, marshy, or floral, depending on the location and time of year the tea was picked.

Oolong tea: Next, you've got your oolong teas, which have been semi-oxidized and roasted, containing medium levels of caffeine. Clay teapots—called *yixing* (ee-SHING) teapots—and other accoutrements were developed by the Chinese and Tawainese especially for these aromatic and complex teas. Chinese oolongs generally tend to have a darker roast and fruitier nature than Taiwanese oolongs, which are generally greener, with a more floral aroma.

Black tea: Black teas are fully oxidized through an intense rolling or tearing process. They're higher in caffeine content than greens and whites but still moderate compared to coffee. Black teas are called red teas in China because the tea, when brewed, has red-colored liquid. Black teas were not widely produced in China until the early nineteenth century.

Pu-erh tea: I would be negligent if I didn't mention a special type of tea you may not have heard of. It's called pu-erh (poo-AIR). Pu-erh teas are aged for a number of years under humid conditions. They have an earthy aroma and a full-bodied flavor, increasing as they age. Pu-erhs come in many forms: loose leaf, compressed into any number of sizes, aged in baskets, bamboo stalks, aged in citrus rinds, and many other forms. Many Chinese drink this tea daily, multiple times a day, to reduce cholesterol levels, decrease blood pressure, and aid digestion.

Tisanes: We tend to call anything "tea" that is made from leaves and steeped in a bag. Technically, however, if it doesn't come from the Camellia sinensis plant, it's not "tea." In other words, if dried flowers, herbs, seeds, or roots (peppermint, camomile, rooibos, for instance) are infused in water, it's what's called a "tisane" and not a "tea."

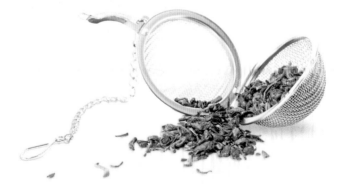

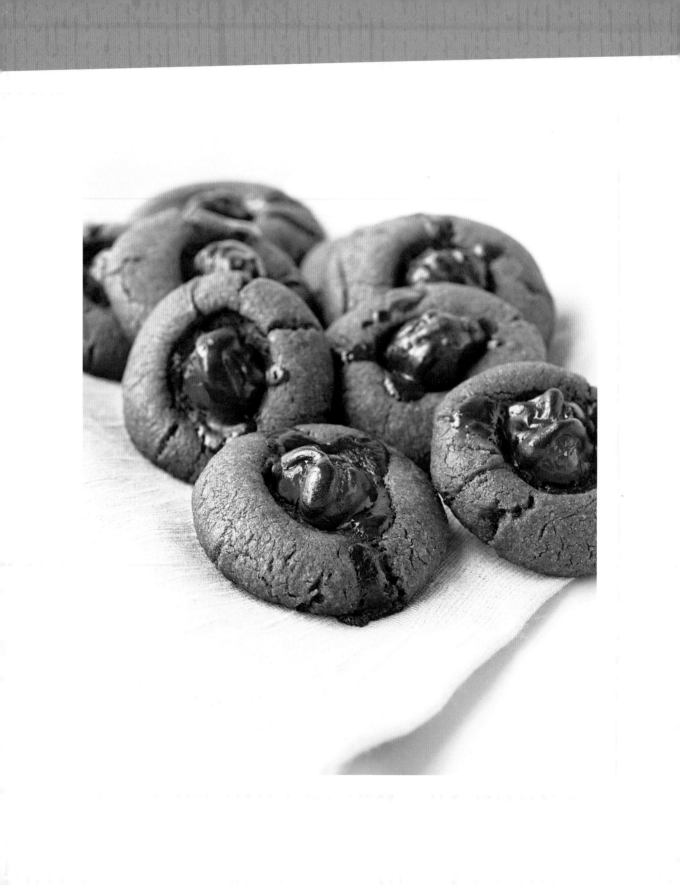

Chocolate Cherry Cookies

I grew up with a father with a chronic sweet tooth, so candy, cakes, and pastries were always in the fridge (or hiding in a drawer somewhere!). Whenever I snuck into the stash, the first thing I would look for was the chocolate-covered cherries. This recipe reminds me of those cookies—and my dad.

1 tablespoon (7 g) ground flaxseed
  (equivalent of 1 egg)
3 tablespoons (30 ml) water
½ cup (112 g) nondairy butter (such as Earth
  Balance), softened
1 cup (200 g) granulated sugar
1½ teaspoons pure vanilla extract
1½ cups (180 g) all-purpose flour
½ cup (60 g) unsweetened cocoa powder
¼ teaspoon baking soda
¼ teaspoon baking powder
¼ teaspoon salt
12 maraschino cherries (reserve juice)
½ cup (88 g) nondairy chocolate chips
  (semisweet or dark)
¼ cup (60 ml) nondairy milk (such as almond,
  soy, rice, hazelnut, hemp, or oat)

DIRECTIONS

Preheat the oven to 350°F (180°C, or gas mark 4).

In a food processor or blender, whip the flax-seed and water together until you have a thick and creamy consistency. This can all be done by hand, but a food processor or blender does a better job in about 1 to 2 minutes. It also makes it creamier than can be done by hand. Transfer the "flax egg" to a medium bowl.

Add the butter and sugar to the bowl with the "flax egg" and using an electric hand mixer, beat until the mixture is creamy and fluffy. Add the vanilla and mix well. Set aside.

In a separate bowl, combine the flour, cocoa, baking soda, baking powder, and salt. Add the dry ingredients to the butter and sugar mixture and stir until just combined. At this point, it may be easier to use your hands because the batter may be too thick for the hand mixer.

Roll the dough into twenty-four 1-inch (2.5 cm) balls and place them 2 inches (5 cm) apart on 2 ungreased baking sheets. Use your thumb to make an indentation in the center of each cookie.

Drain the cherries but reserve the juice. Remove the stems and cut the cherries in half. Place one cherry half into the indentation in each cookie.

Place the chocolate chips and milk in a small saucepan. Stir over low heat until the chocolate is melted. Stir in 4 teaspoons (20 ml) of the cherry juice. Spoon ½ to 1 teaspoon of the melted chocolate over the top of each cherry, covering it completely.

Bake for 10 minutes or until the cookies are firm to the touch and are golden brown on the bottom and cool on a rack.

YIELD: 2 dozen cookies

PER SERVING: 246 Calories; 5g Fat (17.7% calories from fat); 2g Protein; 55g Carbohydrate; 2g Dietary Fiber; 0mg Cholesterol; 103mg Sodium

compassionate cooks' tip

Use the leftover chocolate sauce to make chocolate milk. Just stir it into your favorite nondairy milk.

Cape Brandy Pudding

▶ *Soy-free if using soy-free Earth Balance, oil-free*

This is not a "pudding" in the way we normally think of puddings. It's more of a cake that becomes very moist after adding the syrup. A traditional treat in South Africa, and often referred to as Tipsy Tart, it can be "virginized" by eliminating the brandy.

CAKE/PUDDING

1 cup and 3 tablespoons (280 ml) water, divided

1 cup (175 g) pitted and chopped dates

1 teaspoon baking soda

1 tablespoon (7 g) ground flaxseed

½ cup (112 g) nondairy butter (such as Earth Balance), softened

½ cup (115 g) firmly packed light brown sugar

1 cup (120 g) all-purpose or cake flour

½ teaspoon baking powder

¼ teaspoon salt

½ teaspoon ground cinnamon

¼ teaspoon ground ginger

Pinch of nutmeg

Zest of 1 orange (optional)

½ cup (75 g) chopped walnuts or pecans

SYRUP

⅔ cup (150 g) firmly packed light brown sugar

2 teaspoons nondairy butter (such as Earth Balance)

⅓ cup (80 ml) water

1 teaspoon pure vanilla extract

Pinch of salt

¼ cup (60 ml) brandy (optional)

DIRECTIONS

Preheat the oven to 350°F (180°C, or gas mark 4). Lightly oil an 8 x 8-inch (20 x 20 cm) or a 9 x 9-inch (23 x 23 cm) baking dish.

Bring 1 cup (235 ml) of the water to a boil in a small saucepan. Add the chopped dates and return to a boil, stirring until the dates are soft. Remove from the heat and stir in the baking soda. Mix well and let cool.

In a food processor or blender, combine the ground flaxseed with the remaining 3 tablespoons (45 ml) water and blend for about 1 minute until the mixture becomes thick and gelatinous.

In a bowl, cream together the butter and brown sugar. Add the flax mixture and stir to combine.

To that same bowl, add the flour, baking powder, salt, cinnamon, ginger, nutmeg, orange zest, softened dates, and nuts. Mix together thoroughly.

Pour into the prepared baking dish and bake for 30 minutes, or until a toothpick inserted into the center comes out clean.

While the cake is baking, make the syrup by combining the brown sugar, butter, and water in a saucepan, and simmering over medium-low heat for about 5 minutes, stirring occasionally.

Remove from the heat and stir in the vanilla, salt, and brandy. Pour the warm syrup over the pudding as soon as it is removed from the oven.

YIELD: 6 to 8 servings

PER SERVING: 321 Calories; 16g Fat (44.2% calories from fat); 4g Protein; 42g Carbohydrate; 3g Dietary Fiber; 0mg Cholesterol; 262mg Sodium

WAYS TO INCREASE BROWN AND BLACK FOODS

- Add sliced mushrooms to pasta and salad.

- Choose black sesame seeds instead of the more common tan or white seeds.

- Sprinkle kelp flakes on your salad or in your Better Than Tuna Salad (see *The Vegan Table*).

- Slice nori into small strips and sprinkle on top of salads.

- Incorporate black beans into many dishes (soups, salads, burritos, etc.).

- Add dates to a fruit smoothie.

- Combine brown rice with wild rice for added color and texture.

- Replace brown rice with the gorgeous black Forbidden Rice.

- Drink black tea (I get mine from www.teance.com).

- Snack on black olives or add to salad and pasta dishes.

- Try black quinoa in place of the more common tan quinoa.

- Choose a variety of lentils, including black beluga.

- Incorporate a variety of mushrooms into your diet, including black.

- Add freshly ground black pepper to your dishes.

- Add chopped dates to your oatmeal.

- Choose darker breads when buying sliced bread loaves—the darker, the better.

- When buying chocolate, choose dark. The darker the chocolate, the more antioxidants are present.

- Top your salad with blackberries.

- Keep a container of kelp flakes on the dinner table and use instead of table salt for seasoning foods.

- Add sea vegetables to your next bowl of miso soup.

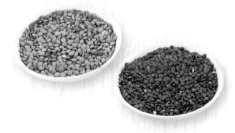

color me THE raINBOW

The idea for this chapter grew out of the desire to offer recipes with no allegiance to one dominant color. After all, the more color *variety* you add to your diet, the more nutrients you consume. Hence, we have our All-Natural Ambrosia (page 246), Couscous and Veggie Medley (page 225), Confetti Macaroni Salad (page 224), Farro and Fresh Vegetable Medley (page 243), Muffuletta Sandwich (page 245), and Southern-Style Succotash (page 237), each of which is packed with a potpourri of color.

Although there is great benefit to pairing certain foods to increase absorption (iron-rich foods with vitamin C; lutein-rich foods with fat; and lycopene-rich foods with heat), I do not believe that eating should be a science experiment. The idea is to eat a great variety of colors as often as possible to achieve maximum nutrition.

However, in terms of flavor, it is true that certain foods pair beautifully together, tantalizing our taste buds while complementing each other in terms of their color. Some of my favorites include the following:

- Potatoes (white, yellow, or purple) and tarragon (green)

- Chickpeas (tan) and mint (green)

- Blueberries (purple) and citrus (yellow, orange, or green)

- Cauliflower (white) and turmeric (orange-yellow)

- Tomatoes (red and orange) and basil (green)

- Root vegetables (variety) and rosemary (green)

- Chocolate (brown) and strawberries (red)—or chocolate and *anything*. (Now you know my weakness.)

Basically, let your senses be your guide. After all, cooking is a fully sensual experience. Consider the following:

- We use our sense of smell to detect delectable aromas (or to warn us of burning rice!).

- Our sense of texture is engaged both tactilely and lingually when we touch and chew food.

- We use our sense of hearing to delight in the sounds of popping corn, sizzling onions, or boiling stew.

- We use our sense of taste to determine preference, for bitter, sour, sweet, and salty.

- And of course, our sense of sight guides us toward gustatory pleasures and optimum health.

advance preparation required

Confetti Macaroni Salad

▶ *Soy-free*

The black poppy seeds add a nice color contrast in this very simple salad perfect for a picnic, quick meal, side dish, or potluck.

1 box (1½ pounds, or 683 g) elbow macaroni
½ red bell pepper, finely diced
½ green bell pepper, finely diced
½ orange bell pepper, finely diced
½ yellow bell pepper, finely diced
3 scallions, chopped
¼ cup (25 g) finely chopped black olives
1 tablespoon (3 g) finely chopped fresh basil
1 cup (225 g) eggless mayonnaise (such as
   Nayonaise, Vegenaise, Wildwood's Garlic Aioli)
2 teaspoons Dijon mustard
Salt and freshly ground pepper, to taste
2 tablespoons (10 g) poppy seeds

DIRECTIONS

Cook the macaroni in salted water according to the package directions until al dente. Drain and set aside.

Meanwhile, combine the bell peppers, scallions, olives, and basil in a bowl and stir to combine.

Add the pasta (it's okay if it's still warm), mayonnaise, and mustard and stir until thoroughly combined. Adjust the seasonings by adding salt and pepper and taste for additional mayonnaise or mustard, adding more if needed. Stir in the poppy seeds.

Cover and refrigerate for at least 2 hours to allow the onion and pepper flavors to permeate the salad.

Serve cold.

YIELD: 8 servings

PER SERVING: 164 Calories; 8g Fat (45.4% calories from fat); 3g Protein; 18g Carbohydrate; 1g Dietary Fiber; 0mg Cholesterol; 46mg Sodium

food lore

Technically, macaroni is any tube-like pasta, though it can take on other shapes as well. Most pastas are not made with eggs, by definition, and macaroni is definitely in that category.

advance preparation required

Couscous and Veggie Medley

▶ *Soy-free, oil-free if omitting the oil*

Enjoy this simple but filling dish on an outing or just as a quick weekday meal.

2 cups (470 ml) vegetable stock

1 teaspoon ground cinnamon

½ teaspoon ground ginger

½ teaspoon ground cumin

¼ teaspoon ground turmeric

1 cup (175 g) uncooked couscous

1 large carrot, finely diced

1 tart apple, unpeeled and diced

1 can (15 ounces, or 420 g) chickpeas

¼ cup (25 g) minced chives or scallions

¼ cup (38 g) raisins or currants

¼ cup (36 g) sunflower seeds (toasted or raw)

1 tablespoon (15 ml) olive oil (optional)

¼ cup (36 ml) fresh lemon juice

½ teaspoon salt, or to taste

½ teaspoon freshly ground pepper, or to taste

DIRECTIONS

In a saucepan, whisk together the stock, cinnamon, ginger, cumin, and turmeric and bring to a boil over high heat. Slowly whisk in the couscous. Stir for 1 minute, cover, remove from the heat, and let sit until all of the liquid has been absorbed, about 15 minutes.

Fluff with a fork and transfer to a large serving bowl, continuing to fluff until the couscous releases all of its steam.

Toss in the carrot, apple, chickpeas, chives, raisins, and sunflower seeds.

In a small jar, combine the olive oil, lemon juice, salt, and pepper. Pour over the couscous and toss until thoroughly blended. Taste and add more salt or lemon juice, if needed.

Chill for at least 4 hours. Bring to room temperature, toss, and adjust the seasonings before serving.

YIELD: 4 to 6 servings

PER SERVING: 321 Calories; 9g Fat (23.9% calories from fat); 10g Protein; 53g Carbohydrate; 7g Dietary Fiber; 0mg Cholesterol; 727mg Sodium

did you know?

Couscous is often mistaken for a "grain," though it is actually small semolina pasta. It whips up in a jiffy, because all you need to do is pour boiling water over the dried couscous and let it soak in the liquid. Although it's typically pretty bland-tasting, it livens up with whatever flavors you add to it.

compassionate cooks' tip

Whole wheat couscous is now available. Look for it in natural foods stores in the bulk section or where the other dry grains are sold.

WHERE DO ANIMALS GET THEIR COLOR?

Now that we understand that all the colors in plants come from phytochemicals, we may take for granted the color of certain animals. As I explained earlier, the phytochemical lutein is what chickens are given to make their flesh and egg yolks yellow; salmon are pink because of the algae they eat; and lobster are only red when boiled because the phytochemicals in their shells become unbound. There are some other things about color and animals you also may not have known.

White Turkeys

Turkeys became the quintessential holiday centerpiece because of a very focused campaign by popular magazine writer Sarah Josepha Hale and because of a successful marketing campaign by the National Turkey Federation. The National Turkey Federation developed a breeding program with the USDA from 1934 to 1941 to develop the "Beltsville White," a turkey with no dark pinfeathers. The breed was introduced commercially in the 1940s and officially recognized by the American Poultry Association in 1951. Bred to produce the most meat, they are also bred so that their carcass has a white color, so that people can have "white meat" versus "dark meat," the natural color of the flesh of dark-feathered, wild birds. Prior to this breeding program, all-white turkeys did not exist. Wild turkeys range in color from brown, gray, and bronze to red, purple, green, copper, and gold—not white.

White Veal

The majority of calves raised to be killed for what is called "veal" are males born to dairy cows. In the United States, more than 700,000 calves are kept and killed for veal each year. Calves kept for both "bob veal" (killed at 21 days young) and "special-fed veal" (killed at 16 to 18 weeks) are confined and tethered in stalls to restrict their movement so they don't develop muscle. They're fed an all-liquid diet, deliberately low in iron to keep their flesh pale.

Pink Flamingos

Although we don't eat flamingos, we manufacture the beauty of those kept in zoos. In the wild, these birds owe their characteristic pink feathers, legs, and face to their diet: carotenoid-rich algae, aquatic plants, and algae-eating crustaceans. An absence of carotenoids in their food results in very pale feathers. Captive flamingos do not eat a carotenoid-rich diet, so zookeepers add synthetic canthaxanthin to their feed to please patrons who want to see a pink-feathered bird.

Goldfish

Even goldfish food manufacturers make specially designed flakes with added carotenoids, such as lycopene, to enhance the color of the fish and make their color more concentrated and bright. The color is in the plants!

Cucumber Salad

▶ *Soy-free, wheat-free, oil-free*

The inspiration for this simple salad was the many Thai restaurants I frequent, which always serve some variation of this dish as a refreshing starter.

2 large cucumbers, seeded and diced, peeling optional

5 purple or red radishes, thinly sliced

1 medium red onion, thinly sliced

¼ cup (60 ml) water

¼ cup (60 ml) rice vinegar, seasoned or regular

1 teaspoon granulated sugar (optional; see below)

¼ to ½ teaspoon crushed red pepper flakes

DIRECTIONS

In a large bowl, combine the cucumbers, radishes, and onion slices.

Add the water, vinegar, sugar, and red pepper flakes, tossing continually to fully coat the vegetables. Let soak for 30 minutes, tossing periodically. Drain and serve.

YIELD: 2 to 4 servings

PER SERVING: 37 Calories; trace Fat (5.6% calories from fat); 1g Protein; 9g Carbohydrate; 2g Dietary Fiber; 0mg Cholesterol; 6mg Sodium

did you know?

Although the flesh of this ancient vegetable, the cucumber (classified botanically as a fruit), contains mostly water and some vitamin C, the skin is worth eating for its insoluble fiber as well as for its potassium and magnesium.

Conventionally grown cucumbers are often coated with wax to prevent bruising during handling and shipping. Plant, insect, animal, or petroleum-based waxes may be used. Organically grown cucumbers tend not to be waxed—just another reason to choose organic, local produce.

compassionate cooks' tip

Seasoned rice vinegar has a little added sugar for sweetness. If you are using seasoned for this dish, you may want to eliminate the sugar; if you are using regular, you might want to add the sugar to sweeten it up.

Carrot and Avocado Salad

▶ *Soy-free, oil-free, wheat-free*

Being a carrot junkie, I often turn to this salad for lunch or a snack. It also makes a great side dish for a refreshing hot-weather meal.

4 or 5 medium carrots, peeled and grated

1 medium ripe avocado, diced

Juice from ½ medium lemon or small orange

Zest from 1 lemon or orange

1 teaspoon balsamic vinegar

Tabasco sauce or hot sauce, to taste

Salt and freshly ground pepper, to taste

3 tablespoons (45 g) toasted sunflower seeds

1 tablespoon (8 g) toasted sesame seeds

DIRECTIONS

Add the carrots, avocado, lemon juice, lemon zest, balsamic vinegar, Tabasco, salt, and pepper to a large bowl. Toss to combine, mashing the avocado as you toss or, if you prefer, tossing gently to keep the avocado intact.

Taste and adjust the seasonings, adding more salt, pepper, and Tabasco, if necessary. Sprinkle the seeds on top and serve immediately.

Alternatively, you may cover and refrigerate it for half an hour or up to a day without the seeds. Just before serving, toss again, adjust the seasonings, and sprinkle the seeds on top.

YIELD: 4 servings

PER SERVING: 205 Calories; 15g Fat (61.6% calories from fat); 4g Protein; 17g Carbohydrate; 6g Dietary Fiber; 0mg Cholesterol; 38mg Sodium

did you know?

Between 1970 and 1986, Americans ate 6 pounds (2.7 kg) of carrots per person per year. However, American consumption of carrots began to take off in 1987, and by 2002 it had reached 11 pounds (5 kg) per person.

compassionate cooks' tips

• Of course, you can grate the carrots by hand, but I have to admit to loving the "grater" blade attachment on my KitchenAid food processor. It takes me all of 60 seconds to grate 5 carrots, and washing up is a snap.

• Toast the seeds in your toaster oven or in a dry sauté pan over low heat. Watch carefully in both instances!

Thai Coconut Soup

▶ *Wheat-free*

This delicious soup was created by one of my favorite chefs, the fabulous Susan Voisin, whose popular blog, *FatFree Vegan Kitchen*, is full of wholesome, flavor-packed recipes and gorgeous photos.

3 cups (705 ml) vegetable stock

1 can (14 ounces, or 395 g) unsweetened coconut milk (light or regular)

2 teaspoons minced fresh ginger

2 teaspoons grated lime zest, plus extra for garnish

2 teaspoons dried lemongrass

½ to 2 teaspoons Thai red curry paste, to taste

12 to 14 ounces (340 to 395 g) extra-firm tofu, cut into small cubes (not silken tofu)

1 can (15 ounces, or 420 g) straw mushrooms, drained and rinsed

2 teaspoons granulated sugar or other sweetener

2 tablespoons (30 ml) tamari soy sauce

1 red bell pepper, sliced into matchstick-size strips

Juice from ½ lime

Cilantro leaves, chopped, for garnish

4 lime wedges, for serving

DIRECTIONS

In a large soup pot, combine the vegetable stock, coconut milk, ginger, 2 teaspoons lime zest, and lemongrass and bring to a boil. Reduce the heat to medium-low and simmer for 5 to 10 minutes.

Add the curry paste ½ teaspoon at a time, stirring well to combine and tasting as you go to make sure you don't make it too spicy. Stir in the tofu, mushrooms, sugar, and tamari, to taste. Simmer for about 10 minutes longer.

Add the red pepper and lime juice, cook for 5 minutes longer to soften the pepper somewhat, season to taste, and remove from the heat. Ladle into 4 bowls, sprinkle with the remaining lime zest and the cilantro leaves, and serve with the lime wedges on the side.

YIELD: 4 servings

SERVING SUGGESTIONS AND VARIATIONS

- Susan noted that because she didn't have fresh or frozen lemongrass, she used dried lemongrass. If you have none of these, she recommends using a couple teaspoons of lemon juice in their stead.
- Other favorite mushrooms may be used in place of the canned straw mushrooms.

PER SERVING: 415 Calories; 30g Fat (61.1% calories from fat); 15g Protein; 28g Carbohydrate; 5g Dietary Fiber; 0mg Cholesterol; 1290mg Sodium

Brazilian Black Bean Stew (*Feijoada*)

▶ *Oil-free if sautéing in water, wheat-free and/or soy-free depending on sausage*

The contrast in spicy and sweet flavors as well as dark and bright colors makes this a fabulous dish for impressing guests.

1 tablespoon (15 ml) oil or water, for sautéing

1 medium yellow onion, chopped

2 cloves garlic, minced

½ pound (225 g) Mexican-spiced vegetarian sausage, cut into half-circles

2 medium garnet or jewel yams, peeled and diced

1 large red bell pepper, diced

2 cans (15 ounces, or 420 g) diced tomatoes

1 small jalapeño pepper, diced

1½ cups (353 ml) water

2 cans (15 ounces, or 420 g) black beans, rinsed and drained

1 mango, peeled, seeded, and cubed

¼ cup (4 g) chopped fresh cilantro, plus extra for garnish

¼ teaspoon salt

DIRECTIONS

Heat the oil in a large soup pot over medium heat, add the onion and garlic, and cook for about 7 minutes until the onion starts to turn translucent.

Add the sausage, yams, bell pepper, diced tomatoes, chile pepper, and water. Bring to a boil, reduce the heat to low, cover, and simmer for 15 minutes or until the yams are tender.

Add the black beans and cook, uncovered, until heated through. Stir in the mango and cilantro and season with salt. Serve hot, garnished with additional cilantro.

YIELD: 4 to 5 servings

PER SERVING: 369 Calories; 7g Fat (17.2% calories from fat); 18g Protein; 60g Carbohydrate; 17g Dietary Fiber; 0mg Cholesterol; 1106mg Sodium

compassionate cooks' tip

Field Roast and Tofurky both make fantastic sausages, the former based on wheat, the latter based on tofu. Both can be found in natural foods stores in the refrigerated sections near the tofu and other vegetarian meats.

food lore

This is a much healthier and tastier version of Brazil's national dish (*feijoada*). After all, the word itself comes from *feijão*, which is Portuguese for "beans."

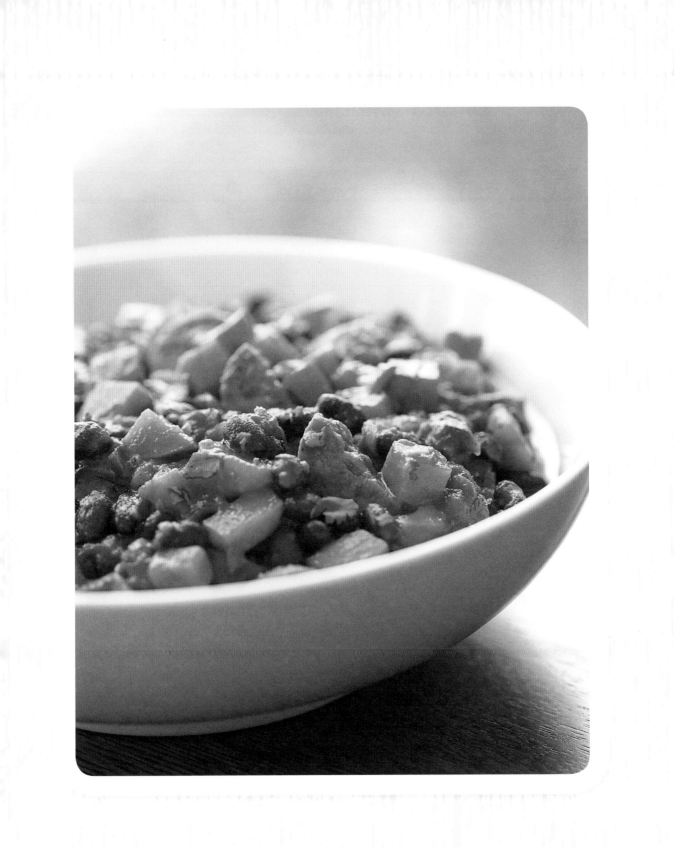

Minestrone with Kale

▶ *Oil-free if using water to sauté, soy-free*

The addition of kale in this classic comfort soup makes it even better, certainly more nutritious, and definitely more colorful!

1 tablespoon (15 ml) oil or water, for sautéing

1 large yellow onion, chopped

2 carrots, finely chopped

4 cloves garlic, finely minced

1 can (15 ounces, or 420 g) diced tomatoes

1 can (15 ounces, or 420 g) white beans (cannellini, Great Northern, navy), rinsed and drained

1 bunch kale (about ¾ pound, or 340 g), stemmed and coarsely chopped

2 tablespoons (8 g) finely chopped fresh parsley

6 cups (1410 ml) water or vegetable stock (or half stock and half water)

2 bay leaves

1 cup cooked (175 g) soup pasta (elbow macaroni, shells, etc.)

Salt and freshly ground pepper, to taste

DIRECTIONS

Heat the oil in a large soup pot over medium heat and add the onion and carrots. Cook, stirring often, until the onion turns translucent and the carrots glisten, about 7 minutes.

Stir in the garlic and cook, stirring, for another minute or so until the garlic begins to smell fragrant. Add the tomatoes and their liquid and cook, stirring occasionally, for about 10 minutes until the tomatoes have cooked down a bit.

Add the beans, kale, parsley, water, and bay leaves. Bring to a boil, reduce the heat to low, cover partially, and simmer for 20 to 30 minutes until the flavors are all incorporated and the kale is tender.

Add the pasta and stir to incorporate. Cook for 5 minutes more, tasting and adjusting the salt and pepper as needed, and then remove from the heat, remove the bay leaves, and serve.

YIELD: 6 servings

PER SERVING: 203 Calories; 4g Fat (16.9% calories from fat); 8g Protein; 36g Carbohydrate; 6g Dietary Fiber; 0mg Cholesterol; 1116mg Sodium

food lore

The Italian word *minestrone* refers to a large, hearty soup. The soup itself is part of what is known in Italy as *cucina povera*—literally "poor kitchen," referring to the necessity of creating dishes based on what was available and in season. Because it has been passed down through the ages, there is no fixed recipe and it lends itself to many variations.

Minted Chickpea Salad

▶ *Soy-free, wheat-free*

This is a delicious "salad" that's hearty enough as a main dish, served atop some shredded green lettuce or as a side to something like the Indian-Style Black Bean and Veggie Burritos (page 238), with which this dish pairs well.

2 cans (15 ounces, or 420 g) cooked chickpeas, rinsed and drained

4 medium tomatoes, seeded and coarsely chopped

1 small red onion, finely chopped

2 or 3 medium cloves garlic, pressed or minced

Juice from 1 lemon

3 to 4 tablespoons (18 to 24 g) minced fresh mint

1 to 2 tablespoons (15 to 30 ml) olive oil

1 cup (70 g) finely shredded green cabbage

1 cup (70 g) finely shredded red cabbage

Salt and freshly ground pepper, to taste

DIRECTIONS

Combine all the ingredients, season as necessary, and let sit for 15 minutes before serving.

YIELD: 4 to 6 servings

PER SERVING: 306 Calories; 9g Fat (24.1% calories from fat); 14g Protein; 47g Carbohydrate; 7g Dietary Fiber; 0mg Cholesterol; 23mg Sodium

compassionate cooks' tip

This salad keeps in the fridge for up to 3 days; after that, it starts to become soggy.

did you know?

If you would like to use dried beans that you cook yourself, you don't have to soak them overnight! You can do a "boil blanch" to speed the process. Bring a large pot of water to a rapid boil. Add your dried beans, cover, and turn off the heat. Let the beans soak for at least an hour and up to two. Next, drain and rinse your beans and return them to the (rinsed) pot. Add the amount of water needed for the beans you're cooking and cook for 2 hours.

food lore

Cicer arietinum, the botanical name for chickpeas, means "small ram," reflecting the fact that the shape of this adorable legume somewhat resembles a ram's head. Chickpeas are also referred to as garbanzo beans, Bengal grams, and Egyptian peas.

Asparagus and Carrots with Walnut Dressing

▶ *Wheat-free, oil-free*

I've used this dressing with other steamed vegetables, such as broccoli and green beans, but I really love it with asparagus and carrots. It's very simple but delicious. This recipe was modified from one in *The Enlightened Kitchen* by Mari Fujii.

10 asparagus spears, thick ends removed

4 carrots, sliced into 1-inch (2.5 cm) matchsticks

¼ to ½ cup (38 to 75 g) raw walnuts

2 teaspoons white/yellow/light miso or
  1 teaspoon red miso

2 tablespoons (30 ml) mirin

2 teaspoons tamari soy sauce

2 tablespoons (30 ml) rice vinegar, regular or
  seasoned

DIRECTIONS

Steam the asparagus and carrots for 5 to 7 minutes until softer but not mushy or roast in a 425°F (220°C, or gas mark 7) oven to the desired doneness. The asparagus should be bright green and the carrots bright orange. Set aside.

Using a food processor or blender, blend together the walnuts, miso, mirin, tamari, and rice vinegar. You can make it nice and creamy (the results of a good blender) or rustic-style, keeping some of the walnut pieces intact. A food processor is more likely to yield a crunchier version.

In a large bowl, combine the carrots and asparagus with the dressing and arrange on a serving plate. Serve hot, warm, or at room temperature.

YIELD: 4 servings

PER SERVING: 184 Calories; 13g Fat (61.3% calories from fat); 5g Protein; 13g Carbohydrate; 5g Dietary Fiber; 0mg Cholesterol; 217mg Sodium

did you know?

Mirin is a kind of rice wine similar to sake but with a lower alcohol content. It has a slightly sweet taste and is a common ingredient in teriyaki sauce.

AN "A" FOR ASPARAGUS

At 4 calories a spear, asparagus is a low-fat, low-calorie, nutrient-dense food. Boasting 33 percent of the Daily Value for folate in just six spears, asparagus also contains high concentrations of vitamin A, vitamin C, and a phytochemical called gluthathione, which has antiviral and anticancer properties.

Go for Glutathione

In fact, according to the National Cancer Institute, asparagus contains more of the antioxidant glutathione than any other fruit or vegetable. Glutathione fulfills numerous functions, including ridding the body of carcinogens, protecting cells and DNA from toxic compounds, participating in boosting immunity, and converting vitamins C and E into usable forms, which may help reduce cataract development in the eye. The tender tips hold the majority of this immune-boosting antioxidant.

Root for Rutin

Rutin is another phytochemical that dwells in asparagus. Lauded for its antioxidant and anti-inflammatory powers, it also strengthens capillary walls. Other sources of rutin include buckwheat, citrus fruits, black tea, and apple peel.

Go for the Green

The green, white, and purple asparagus spears all boast high concentrations of cancer-fighting antioxidants, including vitamins A, C, and E, though the green takes the prize. Consuming a variety is fine, but if you're going for the nutritional gold, go for the green.

What's the Difference?

Green asparagus, an ancient vegetable cultivated by the ancient Egyptians, Greeks, and Romans, is eaten worldwide and contains a high amount of folate, fiber, beta-carotene, and potassium.

White asparagus, also known as *spargel*, is pale because it has been deprived of light. During the growing process, soil is kept mounded around the emerging stalk, which means the plant cannot produce chlorophyll. Without chlorophyll, there is no green color to the stalks. Less bitter than the green variety, it is very popular in the Netherlands, France, Belgium, and Germany.

Purple asparagus, with the addition of the anthocyanin pigment, differs from its green and white counterparts, having high sugar and low fiber levels. First developed in Italy, the purple variety is slightly more bitter than either the white or green but can be used interchangeably in recipes.

Wild Rice and Broccoli

▶ *Wheat-free, soy-free*

This is one of my favorite fall and winter recipes when broccoli is abundant at my local farmers' markets. The chewy black rice contrasts beautifully with the green broccoli and can be served as a main dish, side dish, or light lunch.

3 cups (705 ml) vegetable stock
1 cup (160 g) wild rice, rinsed
½ teaspoon salt, plus more to taste
1 pound (455 g) broccoli florets
⅓ cup (50 g) toasted walnuts, coarsely chopped
⅓ cup (24 g) coarsely chopped fresh herbs, such as parsley, thyme, tarragon, and chives
1 red bell pepper, diced
2 tablespoons (30 ml) fresh lemon juice
1 tablespoon (15 ml) red wine, balsamic, or sherry vinegar
2 cloves garlic, minced
3 tablespoons (45 ml) walnut or olive oil
Freshly ground pepper, to taste

compassionate cooks' tip

A word of warning for people who've never eaten wild rice alone (it's often sold in a combination of different types of rice): it's chewy. Personally, I love the texture, but if you want to tone down the chewiness, you can replace half of the wild rice with long-grain brown.

DIRECTIONS

In a saucepot, bring the stock to a boil over medium heat and then add the rice and ½ teaspoon salt. When the water returns to a boil, reduce the heat to low, cover, and simmer for 45 minutes or until the rice is tender.

Spoon out a few grains and rinse them under cold water. You know they're done when they have split and are tender to the bite (al dente). When you have determined the rice is done, drain and set aside.

Meanwhile, steam the broccoli until just tender, about 5 minutes. Immediately transfer to a bowl with ice-cold water (or rinse in a colander under very cold water), drain, and set aside. (The florets don't need to be in the cold water for more than 3 minutes.) Alternatively, you may heat some olive or walnut oil and sauté the florets for about 7 minutes until the broccoli is cooked and somewhat seared.

In a large bowl, combine the cooked rice, cooked broccoli, toasted walnuts, herbs, and red pepper. Add the lemon juice, vinegar, garlic, and more salt, to taste. Stir in the walnut oil and grind some freshly ground pepper on top. Combine well and taste. Adjust the seasonings as needed. Toss and serve.

YIELD: 3 servings

SERVING SUGGESTIONS AND VARIATIONS
The walnut oil pairs nicely with the broccoli (and walnuts), but olive oil will do in a pinch.

PER SERVING: 479 Calories; 25g Fat (44.8% calories from fat); 15g Protein; 55g Carbohydrate; 8g Dietary Fiber; 0mg Cholesterol; 1383mg Sodium

Southern-Style Succotash

▶ *Wheat-free, oil-free, soy-free if using soy-free Earth Balance and lima beans*

Hominy—corn kernels that have had their germ and hull removed—is readily available in most supermarkets; it is high in calcium and B vitamins.

2 tablespoons (28 g) nondairy butter (such as Earth Balance)

1 large yellow onion, chopped

1 large or 2 small zucchini, diced (but not peeled)

1 package (10 or 12 ounces, or 280 or 340 g) frozen edamame or lima beans, thawed

1 cup (155 g) fresh or frozen corn, thawed

1 red bell pepper, diced

1 can (15 ounces, or 420 g) hominy, rinsed and drained

⅓ cup (80 ml) vegetable stock

½ teaspoon salt

½ teaspoon hot pepper sauce, or to taste

¼ cup (25 g) chopped scallions or chives

DIRECTIONS

Melt the butter in large sauté pan over medium heat. Add the onion and cook and stir for 5 minutes.

Add the zucchini and cook until its flesh becomes more translucent, about 5 minutes.

Add the edamame, corn, and bell pepper. Cook and stir for 5 minutes.

Add the hominy, vegetable stock, salt, and pepper sauce. Simmer for 10 minutes or until most of the liquid has evaporated. Remove from the heat; stir in the scallions. Serve hot.

YIELD: 4 to 6 servings

PER SERVING: 157 Calories; 4g Fat (23.6% calories from fat); 6g Protein; 25g Carbohydrate; 5g Dietary Fiber; 0mg Cholesterol; 335mg Sodium

compassionate cooks' tip

The best way to know when vegetables are done cooking, particularly when using them in a sauté, is to note their color. When the color of the vegetables becomes brighter, that's when they're at their peak of doneness. Overcooking is visible, as the colors become a less bright, and the texture is very soft.

food lore

The word *succotash* is Narragansett for "boiled corn kernels." This type of casserole dish became popular during the Great Depression in the United States and sometimes included a light pie crust on top, making it more like a pot pie. Succotash is a traditional Thanksgiving dish in Pennsylvania and other northeastern states. In Indiana, succotash is made with green beans and corn instead of lima beans.

Indian-Style Black Bean and Veggie Burritos

▶ *Oil-free if sautéing in water, soy-free*

The combination of Southwestern ingredients and Eastern seasonings adds a unique flavor to this burrito.

1 tablespoon (15 ml) oil or water, for sautéing

2 bell peppers (yellow, green, orange, or red), cut into strips

1 large onion, sliced

4 cloves garlic, chopped

1 teaspoon minced fresh ginger

1 sweet potato (or garnet or jewel yam), cut into ½-inch (1.3 cm) cubes

1 teaspoon garam masala

½ cup (120 ml) vegetable stock

1 can (15 ounces, or 420 g) black beans, drained and rinsed

Salt and freshly ground pepper, to taste

1 cup (165 g) cooked brown basmati rice

1 head romaine lettuce, shredded

Pineapple Mango Chutney (page 74) or salsa of your choice

4 large burrito-size whole wheat tortillas

DIRECTIONS

Heat the oil in a large sauté pan. Sauté the bell peppers, onion, garlic, and ginger over medium heat for 7 to 10 minutes, stirring frequently, until the peppers and onion are soft.

Add the sweet potato and garam masala and mix well. Add the stock, and cover. Cook over medium-low heat for 10 to 15 minutes or until the potato is tender.

At the very end of the cooking time, add the beans and stir to combine. Cook for 5 minutes longer and season with salt and pepper.

Spoon the vegetable and bean mixture, rice, lettuce, and chutney evenly down the center of a tortilla and then roll it up. Serve immediately.

YIELD: 4 servings

SERVING SUGGESTIONS AND VARIATIONS

To make this dish even prettier, use tomato or spinach tortillas instead of whole wheat; or use a combination and serve them together on a platter.

PER SERVING: 780 Calories; 17g Fat (18.4% calories from fat); 20g Protein; 146g Carbohydrate; 19g Dietary Fiber; 0mg Cholesterol; 900mg Sodium

food lore

Garam masala is Hindi for "spicy mixture." It's basically a spice mixture found in the spice aisle of grocery stores that typically contains peppercorns, cloves, bay leaves, cumin, cardamom, nutmeg, and anise.

compassionate cooks' tip

Warm the tortillas to make them more pliable.

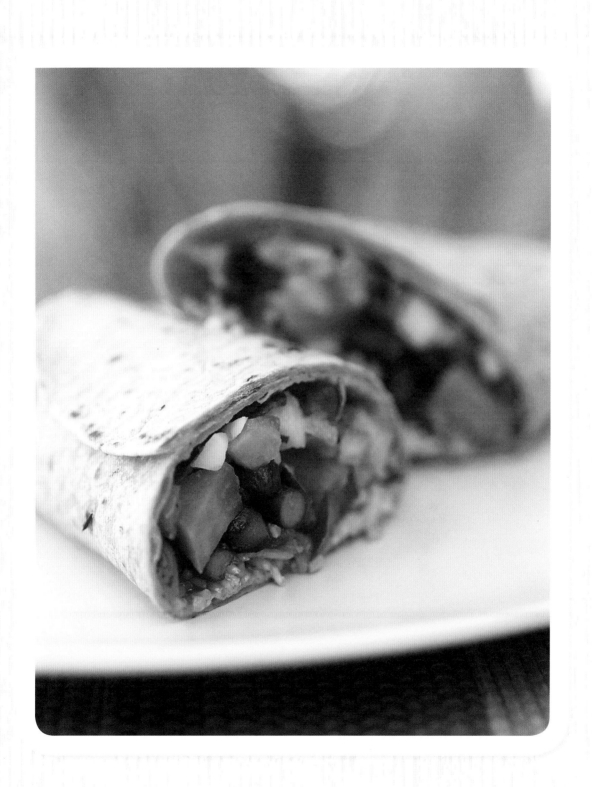

HOW TO ROLL A BURRITO

1. The first thing to know is to avoid overfilling your burrito. Too much filling, and it's difficult to roll.

2. Make sure your beans are drained so you're not adding unnecessary liquid. Use a slotted spoon if taking them right from the water you heated them in and give it a couple of shakes before spooning them onto the tortilla.

3. Use the large 14- or 16-inch (35.5 or 40.5 cm) burrito tortillas rather than the smaller taco-size ones. They make rolling foolproof.

4. Make sure the tortilla is warm and pliable. You may heat tortillas in the toaster oven, over a steamer, on a hot skillet, over an open flame (via a grill or gas burner), or in the microwave.

5. Place the various fillings (beans, salsa, guacamole, lettuce, tomatoes) evenly across the center of the tortilla. The filling should be in the center and not close to any of the edges.

6. Fold the bottom of the tortilla up so that it totally or mostly covers the filling.

7. Fold the left or right side of the burrito in and slightly downward. You want to cover half or two-thirds of the tortilla's width with this movement.

8. Fold the other side in the same fashion, again pushing on it a bit to spread the filling out.

9. While holding the ends of the burrito, roll or flip the burrito over, folding the top flap as you do.

10. Eat or wrap in foil and heat on a griddle or in the oven.

"Sloppy Col" Sandwich

▶ *Soy-free, oil-free*

This is a summer staple in the Patrick-Goudreau household because it is so easy to make and so fresh. Vary the veggies based on your own preferences.

½ cup (112 g) hummus, store-bought or homemade (see recipe in *The Vegan Table*)
1 fresh baguette or 2 to 4 fresh whole wheat rolls
1 ripe avocado, seeded and sliced
2 roasted red bell peppers, sliced
1 bunch alfalfa sprouts
2 or 3 carrots, shredded
2 tomatoes, sliced
1 cup (20 g) mixed salad greens
Salt and freshly ground pepper, to taste

DIRECTIONS

Spread some hummus on the bread—or if you prefer, use the avocado as your spread, or both! If you use the hummus as the spread, you can still add the avocado as one of the sandwich fillers.

Create your sandwich. Add the peppers, sprouts, carrots, tomatoes, salad greens, and any other ingredients you wish. No need to measure anything—just pile on the veggies! It's that easy.

Sprinkle on some salt and grind some pepper on top of the ingredients and repeat to make another sandwich.

YIELD: 2 to 4 sandwiches

SERVING SUGGESTIONS AND VARIATIONS

• Use focaccia or pita bread instead of a baguette.
• Add pesto instead of hummus and drizzle a little balsamic vinegar over the veggies.
• Add Garlic Aioli, a delicious eggless mayonnaise made by Wildwood, or Vegenaise or Nayonaise.

PER SERVING: 258 Calories; 12g Fat (39.2% calories from fat); 8g Protein; 35g Carbohydrate; 9g Dietary Fiber; 0mg Cholesterol; 273mg Sodium

did you know?

Red bell peppers contain more vitamin C than oranges; they're in the top ten for beta-carotene content; and they're one of the best sources for the carotenoids lutein, zeaxanthin, and beta-cryptoxanthin. Red peppers, like tomatoes, also contain lycopene, a carotenoid whose consumption has been inversely correlated with prostate cancer and cancers of the cervix, bladder, and pancreas.

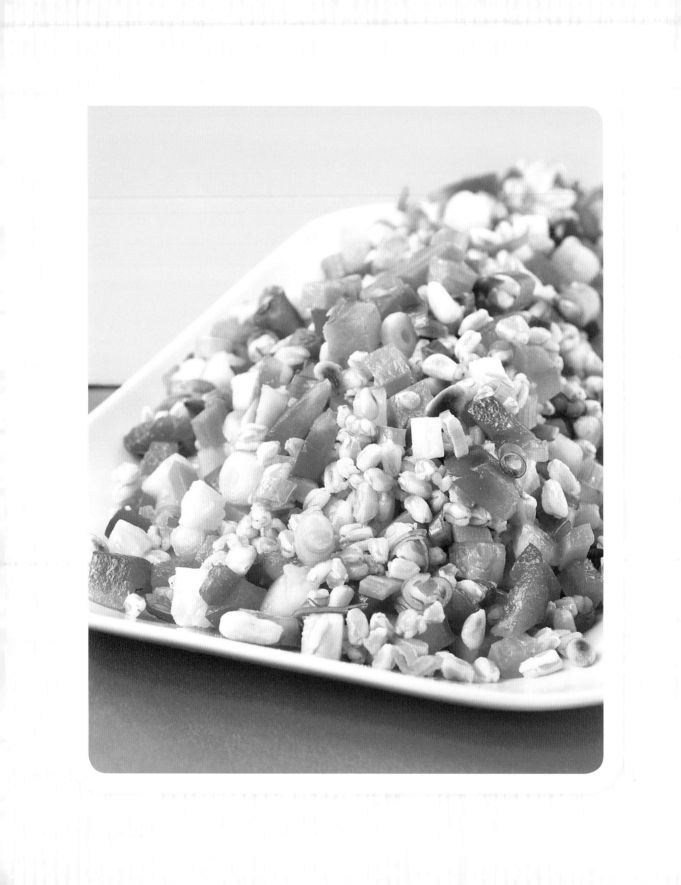

Farro and Fresh Vegetable Medley

▶ *Wheat-free, soy-free*

Thanks to podcast listeners Chris Courtney and Teje Court, I am able to share this recipe with you. Chris and Teje lived in Italy for several years, where they fell in love with this hearty and nutty-tasting grain and graced me with not only this recipe but also several bags of farro direct from Italy.

2 cups (368 g) uncooked farro or barley
5 cups (1175 ml) water or vegetable stock
1 cup (150 g) diced bell pepper (red, orange, or yellow)
1 cup (130 g) diced carrot (about 4 or 5 carrots)
1 cup (135 g) diced cucumber, unpeeled
1 cup (100 g) chopped scallions (about 6 scallions using both white and green parts)
½ to ¾ cup (68 to 100 g) toasted pine nuts
½ cup (32 g) finely chopped parsley
½ cup (32 g) finely chopped mint
1 to 2 tablespoons (15 to 30 ml) balsamic vinegar
¼ to ⅓ cup (60 to 80 ml) olive oil
Juice of 1 or 2 small lemons, divided
Salt and freshly ground pepper, to taste

DIRECTIONS

In a 3- or 4-quart (3.3 or 4.4 L) saucepan, combine the farro and water, and bring to a boil over high heat. Reduce the heat to low and simmer without stirring for 35 to 45 minutes until the stock is absorbed. Remove from the heat.

Meanwhile, in a large bowl, add the bell pepper, carrot, cucumber, scallions, pine nuts, parsley, and mint. Stir to combine. Add the vinegar, olive oil, the juice of 1 lemon, and salt and pepper, to taste. Add the cooked farro, taste, and add more lemon juice and salt, if necessary.

Serve right away or the next day. Yummers!

YIELD: 8 servings

SERVING SUGGESTIONS AND VARIATIONS

Use one finely chopped red onion in place of the scallions.

PER SERVING: 331 Calories; 16g Fat (41.4% calories from fat); 9g Protein; 42g Carbohydrate; 9g Dietary Fiber; 0mg Cholesterol; 638mg Sodium

food lore

Farro is one of the ancient cereal crops of the Mediterranean region, along with wheat, spelt, and barley. Because it grows well even in poor soil and is resistant to fungus, farro grows wild (an archaeological site in modern-day Israel dated some from 17,000 BCE), in addition to being a domesticated crop. The earliest evidence of domesticated farro was found at an archaeological site dated around 7700 BCE, near Damascus in modern-day Syria.

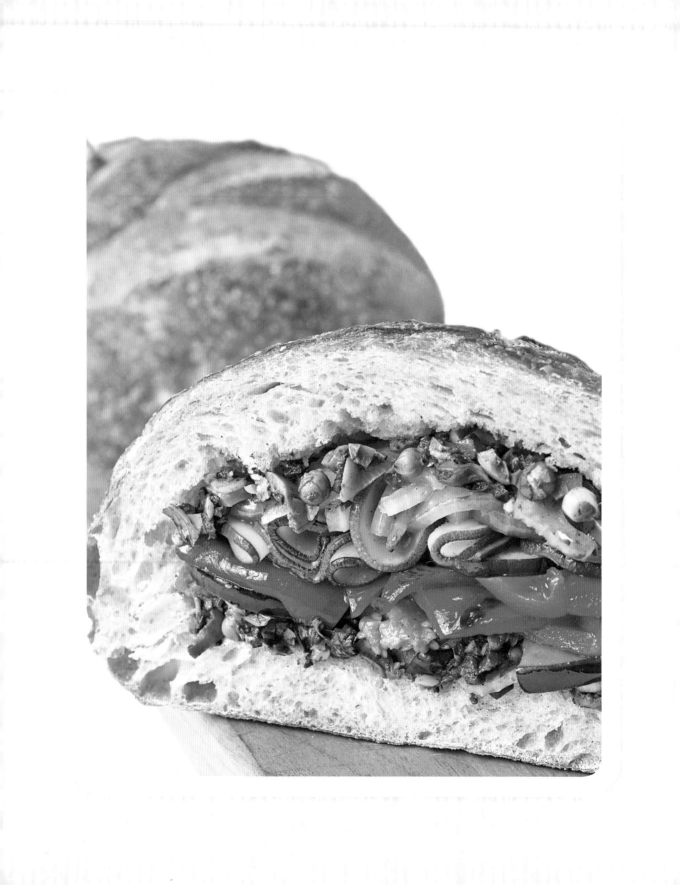

advance preparation required

Muffuletta Sandwich

▶ *Soy-free*

This is an animal-friendly version of the New Orleans signature sandwich.

SANDWICH

1 Italian globe eggplant, cut into ⅓-inch (8 mm)-thick rounds

1 large zucchini, cut into ⅓-inch (8 mm)-thick rounds

1 large sweet onion, thinly sliced

2 red or yellow bell peppers, stemmed, seeded, and quartered

2 large tomatoes, sliced

Olive oil, for brushing

1 round loaf hearty French or Italian bread

OLIVE SALAD

2 cups (200 g) green olives, pitted

½ cup (50 g) kalamata olives, pitted

3 tablespoons (45 ml) brine from olives

2 tablespoons (17 g) capers

4 cloves garlic, thinly sliced

3 stalks celery, thinly sliced

1 tablespoon (4 g) finely chopped fresh parsley

1 tablespoon (3 g) dried oregano

1 teaspoon crushed red pepper flakes

⅓ cup (80 ml) olive oil

3 tablespoons (45 ml) red wine vinegar

3 scallions, finely chopped

Salt and freshly ground pepper, to taste

DIRECTIONS

Lightly oil a baking sheet and preheat the oven to 425°F (220°C, or gas mark 7) to roast the vegetables.

To make the sandwiches, brush all sides of the eggplant, zucchini, onion, bell peppers, and tomatoes with olive oil. Arrange them on the baking sheet and roast in the oven for 15 to 30 minutes, or until browned and tender. Check the tomatoes after 5 minutes because they cook quickly and may fall apart when you try to remove them from the baking sheet.

If you choose to grill the vegetables, place them on the grill after brushing them with oil and grill for 5 to 7 minutes on both sides until charred and tender.

Meanwhile, to make the olive salad, add the green olives and kalamata olives to a food processor and pulse until finely chopped. Transfer to a large bowl and add the olive brine, capers, garlic, celery, parsley, oregano, and red pepper flakes. Toss to combine.

In a small bowl, whisk together the olive oil, vinegar, scallions, and salt and pepper, to taste. Drizzle over the olive salad ingredients and stir to thoroughly combine, making sure all the vegetables are coated. (Use right away or store in the refrigerator for up to a week to intensify the flavor.)

Cut the loaf of bread in half lengthwise and remove some of the soft center to provide room for the filling. Spoon the olive salad on both sides of the bread sandwiching the layer of roasted vegetables in between.

For best results, wrap the sandwich tightly in foil and refrigerate for at least 1 hour and up to 3 hours before serving.

Cut into 4 to 6 wedges and serve.

YIELD: 4 to 6 servings

PER SERVING: 439 Calories; 21g Fat (41.3% calories from fat); 9g Protein; 56g Carbohydrate; 8g Dietary Fiber; 0mg Cholesterol; 1188mg Sodium

All-Natural Ambrosia

▶ *Soy-free, wheat-free, oil-free*

If you're at all familiar with the original version of this dish, I urge you to block it from your mind and turn instead to this one: delicious, healthful, and colorful.

1 ½ cups (233 g) fresh pineapple, diced

1 large banana, sliced

1 ½ cups (240 g) organic red or green seedless grapes, halved or whole

⅔ cup (46 g) shredded raw coconut

2 tablespoons (30 ml) freshly squeezed orange juice

1 tablespoon (5 g) fresh orange zest

½ cup (75 g) walnut pieces, toasted

1 large banana, puréed

½ teaspoon pure vanilla extract

DIRECTIONS

In a large bowl, combine the pineapple, sliced banana, grapes, coconut, orange juice, orange zest, and walnuts. Set aside or cover and refrigerate if you are not serving it right away. Do not add the puréed banana until you're ready to serve.

When ready to serve, add the puréed banana and vanilla and toss until coated and combined. Serve in pretty glass bowls.

YIELD: 4 servings

PER SERVING: 266 Calories; 15g Fat (46.4% calories from fat); 6g Protein; 33g Carbohydrate; 4g Dietary Fiber; 0mg Cholesterol; 4mg Sodium

food lore

In ancient Greek mythology, ambrosia was the magical food of the gods ("nectar" was the magical drink), and it would confer ageless immortality upon whoever consumed it. The word *ambrosia* means "fragrant" or "delicious," but I must admit I don't think the gods would have been eager to eat what became a popular dish in the United States, laden as it is with artificial colors, fat-saturated heavy cream, sour cream, whipping cream, and marshmallows and dependent upon canned pineapple, canned maraschino cherries, and canned oranges. With those ingredients, I suppose it does challenge mortality. If you can survive the saturated fat, sugar, and cholesterol, you're immortal!

FINDING NATURAL FOOD COLORING

Many years ago, I was conducting a supermarket tour with a father of three children. We had filled his shopping cart with an abundance of colorful fruits and veggies, and he paused and said, "I'm so struck by the fact that the color in my cart is because of all the produce. It's usually from the boxes of cereal I buy for the kids."

Color is a highly marketable element. "Food" manufacturers know this and they exploit it. I say "food" in quotes because I don't consider artificial flavorings, artificial colorings, and processed ingredients "food." Food is real. Food is whole. Food is nutrient-rich, not nutrient-poor. And nutrient-poor products in bright colors are marketed to children, in particular—not only in terms of packaging but also in terms of artificial food coloring. In fact, studies have found that children may consume 50 to 300 milligrams of artificial coloring in a day.

Natural versus Artificial Coloring

There are two types of food dyes: those derived from natural sources and those that are artificially manufactured. The latter are mostly coal-tar derivatives made from chemical compounds. The Food and Drug Administration (FDA) is responsible for regulating all color additives used in the United States, whether they are natural or synthetic or used for food, paints, cosmetics, textiles/clothing, inks, or medicines.

Synthetic color additives are not only cheaper than natural dyes, but they are also more intense in their hue and neutral in their flavor. They are the center of controversy as to whether they are harmful. Some camps say they are; some camps say they aren't. Although the jury is still out, I just prefer to seek out real food as much as possible, including dyes made from plants rather than laboratories or animal products. For example, cochineal and carmine, the cryptic names on ingredients lists, are actually colorings derived from ground-up beetles.

Natural Food Dyes

Plenty of natural food colorings are available.

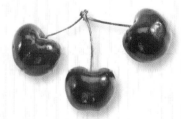

- Some natural red colors are derived from cherry and beet juices.
- Annatto is a red waxy substance from the seed of a shrub in Central America also used to make natural red dyes.
- Saffron is used to create a yellow color.
- Indigo, a blue color derived from the indigo plant, is one of the best-known natural colorings and has been used for centuries.
- Caramel color, used in sauces, gravies, baked goods, and (eek!) sodas, is produced by heating sugar and other carbohydrates under controlled conditions.

Chocolate, Banana, and Almond Butter Panini

▶ *Oil-free and soy-free if using soy-free Earth Balance*

I'm of the school of thought that believes fruit is awesome and warm fruit is even better. You don't need a panini maker to enjoy these, but you'll most likely want one after you experience the joy that is fruit panini.

½ cup (130 g) almond butter

4 slices thinly sliced bread, crusts removed

½ cup (90 g) nondairy semisweet or dark chocolate chips

1 banana, sliced into flat strips or cut into rounds

Light cooking spray or 2 tablespoons (28 g) nondairy butter (such as Earth Balance), divided

DIRECTIONS

Preheat your panini maker, if using. Spread a generous amount of almond butter on 1 side of each of the 4 bread slices. Sprinkle the chocolate chips on top of the almond butter on 2 of the 4 slices so they stick.

Lay the banana strips on top of the chocolate chips. Carefully place the 2 slices with almond butter on top of the 2 pieces of bread that have the chocolate chips and banana and press gently to close.

Lightly spray your preheated panini maker with a little cooking oil to ensure the sandwiches don't stick. Place 1 or 2 sandwiches (depending on the size of your machine) in the panini maker, press down, and cook for 4 minutes.

If you aren't using a panini maker, melt 1 tablespoon (14 g) of the nondairy butter in a medium sauté pan over medium heat. Place 1 sandwich in the pan, place a flat heavy object on top, such as a cutting board, and cook for about 3 minutes on each side. (Stay close so they don't burn.) The chocolate should be melted.

Remove from the pan and repeat with the second sandwich and remaining 1 tablespoon (14 g) butter.

Slice each sandwich in half on the diagonal and serve immediately while they're nice and warm!

YIELD: 2 sandwiches

SERVING SUGGESTIONS AND VARIATIONS

A countertop grill works as well as a panini maker.

PER SERVING: 824 Calories; 55g Fat (56.3% calories from fat); 17g Protein; 79g Carbohydrate; 8g Dietary Fiber; 0mg Cholesterol; 295mg Sodium

did you know?

The singular version of the Italian word for "sandwich" is *panino*, and the plural is *panini*.

SIMPLE WAYS TO ADD COLOR

- Keep fruits and vegetables—fresh and frozen—stocked and in sight.

- Chop vegetables in advance and store them in containers in your fridge for easy access.

- Choose truly natural (no preservatives) juice instead of coffee or soda.

- Choose leaf lettuce with the darkest green or red leaves for an added nutritional boost.

- Add chopped fruit (fresh or dried) to cereal, nondairy yogurt, pancakes, muffins, toast, bagels, or even a sandwich!

- Snack on fresh chopped carrots, celery, broccoli, cauliflower, and bell peppers. If you don't chop them in advance yourself, purchase them at a salad bar.

- Add leafy green veggies, such as kale and chard, to all your soups.

- Add fresh chopped herbs to soups, salads, and sandwiches.

- Keep dried fruit (apricots, dates, or raisins) for a quick snack at home or work.

- Add grapes, pineapple, grated carrots, or other vegetables to such salads/sandwiches as Better Than Tuna Salad and Better Than Chicken Salad (in *The Vegan Table*).

- Whip up a stir-fry several nights a week with a variety of vegetables. Change it up by varying the sauce.

- Shop at your local farmers' market or produce stand and choose produce you've never tried before.

- Add vegetables to pasta dishes.

- Add fresh greens, carrots, and tomatoes to homemade and canned soup.

- Add fresh vegetables to your pizza.

- Invest in a juicer and make regular juices from carrots, apples, beets, ginger, pears, and oranges. (My favorite!)

- Find inspiration from a box of crayons: pack as many colors as you can into one container by taking a basic spinach salad and adding radicchio, different color bell peppers, tomatoes, carrots, mandarin oranges, raspberries, and blueberries. Top with raspberry vinaigrette.

- Instead of ice cream, make one of my favorite frozen treats. (See Frozen Banana Dessert on page 99.)

Strawberries with Lavender Syrup

▶ *Oil-free, wheat-free, soy-free*

This dish is a summer delight, especially if you get your strawberries and lavender from your backyard, like I do, or from your local farmers' market.

⅓ cup plus ½ cup (165 g) granulated sugar,
    divided, or less, to taste
1 teaspoon grated lemon zest
½ cup (120 ml) water
2 tablespoons (40 g) agave nectar
2 teaspoons dried culinary lavender
3 pints (870 g) strawberries, sliced
5 mint leaves, finely minced

did you know?

Find dried culinary lavender where the other dried herbs and spices are in your grocery store. If you opt for fresh culinary lavender, you'll want to double the amount.

Lemon juice is essential for bringing out the color of the cooked potatoes, so don't skip this step!

DIRECTIONS

Combine ⅓ cup (65 g) of the sugar and lemon zest in a small bowl. Blend well and either use right away or store in the refrigerator in a covered container.

In a saucepan over medium-high heat, bring the remaining ½ cup (100 g) sugar, water, agave nectar, and lavender to a boil, stirring until the sugar dissolves. Reduce the heat to medium and simmer until the lavender flavor is detectable, about 5 minutes.

Strain the syrup into a small bowl or store in a container, cover, and let stand at room temperature. Reheat the syrup before using.

When ready to serve, place the strawberries in large serving bowl. Pour the warmed syrup over the berries and stir to coat. Divide the syrup-covered strawberries among 8 plates or bowls, sprinkle with the lemon sugar and finely minced mint, and serve immediately.

YIELD: 8 servings

SERVING SUGGESTIONS AND VARIATIONS

- Strawberries go well with bubbly. Serve on a special occasion with a glass of Champagne and toast to your health.
- Decrease the amount of sugar if it is too sweet for you.

PER SERVING: 122 Calories; trace Fat (1.8% calories from fat); trace Protein; 31g Carbohydrate; 2g Dietary Fiber; 0mg Cholesterol; 2mg Sodium

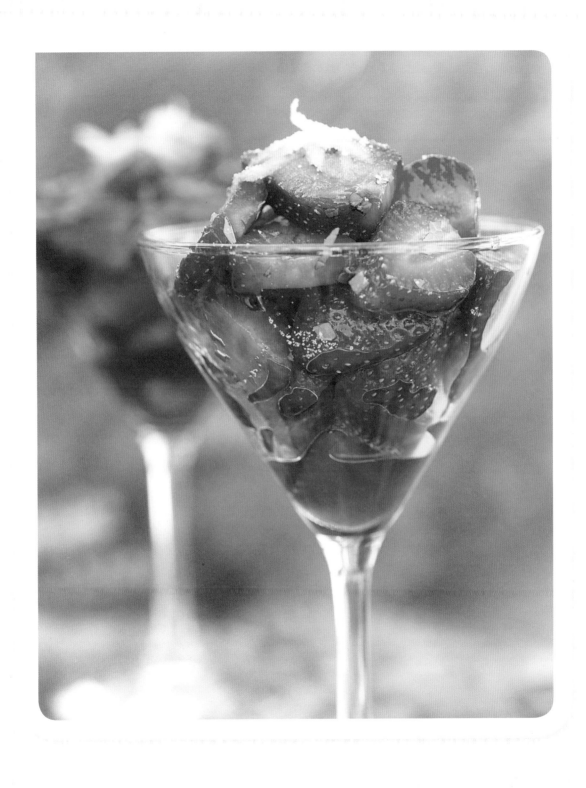

RESOURCES AND RECOMMENDATIONS

RESOURCES

Agave Nectar

Madhava
www.madhavasagave.com

Eggless Mayonnaise

Wildwood's Garlic Aioli
www.wildwoodfoods.com

Vegenaise
www.followyourheart.com

Find a Farmer's Market Near You

www.localharvest.org

Hijiki and Sea Vegetables

Eden Foods, Inc.
www.edenfoods.com

Nondairy Yogurt

Soymilk-based

Wildwood
www.wildwoodfoods.com

Whole Soy & Co.
www.wholesoyco.com

Trader Joe's brand
www.traderjoes.com

Rice milk–based

Ricera
www.ricerafoods.com

Coconut milk–based

So Delicious
www.turtlemountain.com

Saffron Extract

Supreme Spice
www.supremespice.com

Tea

www.teance.com

Vegan Marshmallows

Sweet & Sara
www.sweetandsara.com

Dandies Candies
www.dandiescandies.com

RECOMMENDATIONS

Supplements

Visit www.compassionatecooks.com to view and purchase the Dr. Fuhrman line of supplements, including multivitamins, DHA supplements, and more.

Kitchen Items

People ask me all the time what my favorite kitchen items are. Please visit www.compassionatecooks.com and click on "Buy Kitchen Items & Books" under "Shop" to find all my recommendations at my Amazon store, including those I name below.

Favorite Food Processor

KitchenAid
www.kitchenaid.com

Favorite Blender

Vitamix is my absolute favorite, but if it's too pricey for you, then I recommend KitchenAid.
www.vitamix.com
www.kitchenaid.com

ACKNOWLEDGMENTS

Thanks to everyone at Fair Winds Press for creating another beautiful manifestation of my vision. I knew a cookbook based on color would be gorgeous in your very capable hands, and I was right. And now, we officially have a trilogy.

Being part of a movement dedicated to saving human and nonhuman lives and improving the world is incredibly gratifying and most definitely humbling. I'm so grateful to do this work alongside so many compassionate individuals and organizations. It's been an absolute joy to teach for Dr. McDougall's Wellness Program for so many years. Not only are Mary and John wonderfully supportive, but their staff is a delight to work with. (Thank you for your love and patience each month, Tiffany!) More than that, the folks who come through their program—who I have the privilege of teaching—are some of the most open, friendly, and generous people I've ever met. Their eagerness to learn and change is one of the reasons I have hope in this world.

Thanks so much to Patti Breitman for guiding me yet again, to VegNews Magazine for including me as part of your family of columnists, and to Dr. Michael Greger for your awesome fact-checking!

Each and every one of my recipes is tested by a number of people once I think it is at the "done" stage. I'm so grateful to everyone who generously gave their time and feedback to make sure the recipes were perfect. The enthusiasm with which the testers prepared these recipes and the care with which they combed them for accuracy and readability led to make this book what it is. I was particularly impressed with those who would receive my recipes, test them despite having to use ingredients they weren't fond of (but not tell me until afterwards), and then declare how much the liked the recipe—even though they didn't think they would. You gotta love that kind of commitment and openness! Thank you to:

Brian Walsh, Marie Levey-Pabst, Liz Zeigler, Chastity, Trish Sutton, Valerie Douchette, Cheryl Crain, Janet Frick, Cheryl Crain, Valerie Douchette, Janet Frick, Lori Moffei, Terri Elder, Diana Kaempfer, Rose Glover, Jennifer Garish, Faith Gundran, Marla Rose, Brighde Reed, Marika Collins, and Carrie Dawley.

Wonderful as all of these testers were, I would be negligent if I didn't make special mention of three in particular who were Superheroes throughout the process: Ruth Boogert, Jenny Howard, and Barbara Lyons, who were testing upwards of five recipes per week—consistently. To boot, Barbara's feedback was accompanied by gorgeous photos of each of the dishes she tested. (Search for Color Me Vegan at flickr.com.)

Because of the support of a number of unbelievably generous people, I'm able to keep up with the many projects and emails at Compassionate Cooks.

Amanda Mitchell is my angel, answering each and every email with thoroughness and joy, managing the membership program, providing research when necessary, being the point person for Compassionate Cooks volunteers, adroitly directing communications, writing and designing the monthly newsletters, and being my biggest support (next to my hubby, of course).

Megan Storms has taken a huge load off of my shoulders by managing the compassionatecooks. com website. Adding pages, content, graphics, links, audio, video, and more, Megan has quite literally freed up several hours of each week for me to devote to writing. She saved me from facing the dreaded alternative of letting the website get stale, which is the last thing I wanted to do. You are my hero, Megan. Thank you!

Tami Hiltz is our Oregon-based, one-person fulfillment house! Each and every order placed through compassionatecooks.com is sent out by Tami. Making trips to the post office, stocking up on shipping supplies, ensuring inventory is in stock are just a few of the things Tami takes care of—and always with immense pleasure and joy. Around here, she's known as St. Tami.

Jennifer Stadtmiller is our uber lovely Compassionate Cooks Facebook Fan Page manager, keeping things interesting and community-oriented over at the popular networking site.

Juliet Lynn designed our beautiful *The Vegan Table* website (vegantable.com) as well as the website dedicated to *Color Me Vegan* (colormevegan.com).

Though I'm taking an indefinite hiatus from my own cooking classes, I did continue to teach while I was writing *Color Me Vegan* and have to thank Lori Patotzka, Matt Props, Megan McClellan, Jared Greer, and Pam Webb for being reliable, dedicated assistants and Ryan Thibodaux and Poppy Nguyen for prepping all those vegetables!

Aaron Weinstein—I wouldn't have a beautiful brochure if it weren't for Aaron's generosity and talents. Taking care of all my design needs, Aaron spends his rare off-hours making sure Compassionate Cooks' materials are visually appealing and as perfect as can be.

Stephen and Danielle Tschirhart generously take care of my printing needs, including spending their own money to have my brochure printed professionally. Amazing.

Eric Zamost—with generosity and humility, Eric duplicates my podcast sampler CDs so people can distribute them others to inspire them to listen and learn. Always making sure they're delivered on time an in tact, Eric is always a calming presence—even when I make requests on ridiculously short notice.

Blake Wiers—one of those gifts of marriage, Blake was my husband's college roommate and now I get to benefit not only from his friendship but from his filmmaking and editing prowess as well. Blake generously spent countless hours choosing video clips, photos, and audio for my "Colleen-in-a-Nutshell" video.

Thanks also to Asae Dean for managing my (now-defunct-by-choice) MySpace page, Natasha Prince for helping out with research, Cheryl Foley for managing our fantastic partnerships and sponsorships, Diane Mayo for many months of newsletter content-gathering, Grace Parker-Guerrero for keeping my administrative house in order, Kelly Kramer for doing the same and for providing top-notch kitty love to Simon, Schuster, and Cassandra. Ditto Michael Scribner. Damnit I miss you!

My special Compassionate Cooks Members provide much-needed support to our podcast and projects. Thank you Heide Allebach, Stephanie Andrews, Mick Barr, Leona Llamoy Cunningham III, Jessica Deschaines, Tia Doane, Stephanie Noelle Garza, Chelsea Hassler, Beth Henderson, Michelle Howe, Kaitlin Jones, Marlinda Karo, Jennifer Kearns, Laura Keddy, Jamie Koplin, David Kwon, Melissa Leitch, Peter and Eric Lu of peacefood cafe nyc, Christopher Lutz, Michelle Lynde, Jennifer Meara, Colleen Molenda, Sara Newton, Kimberly Pembleton, Danielle Phillips, Jennifer Rasper, Michaela Ryann Riley and Ian Riley, Kimberly Roemer, Sheila Roering, Mary Spears, Megan and Eric Storms, Melissa Tedrowe, Laura Valle, Mary Wendt, and Shawn Zurek.

Blessed to have so many supportive and loving friends and family, I am especially thankful for Diane Miller, Cadry Nelson, David Busch, Kenda Swartz, Michael Scribner, Chris Marco, Shad Clark, Kristen Schwarz, Tami Wall, Cheri Larsh Arellano, Mark Arellano, John Keathley, Randy Lind, Cathleen Young, Deborah Underwood, Robin Brande, Rae Sikora, and family: mom Arlene, dad John, sister-in-love Jen, and parents by marriage, Mary Jane and Paul Goudreau. Everyone else I hold dear has either already been mentioned here or is in my heart.

Living with animals is a gift, and my cats fill every moment of my life with joy and awe. Though we still mourn the loss of Simon, our boy of almost 16 years, we treasure each second with his brother Schuster; he is the light of my life. We were also blessed to make Cassandra part of our home in the latter years of her life and miss her sweet presence every day. Our newest bean, Sir Charles, brightens up our home and our lives, and we look forward to many years with Schustie's new companion.

Last but in every way *first*, I am most grateful to my beloved husband David Goudreau—my greatest friend and biggest support. He helps me in every way and always with patience, love, and devotion. There is nothing that gives me more pleasure than making him laugh and seeing him smile.

Che importa la ricchezza
Se alfine è rifiorita La felicità!
O sogno d'or
Poter amar così!

ABOUT THE AUTHOR

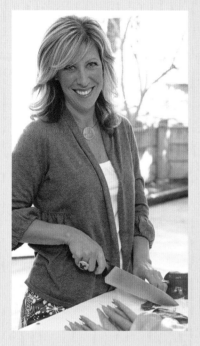

Colleen Patrick-Goudreau is the author of two best-selling cookbooks, *The Joy of Vegan Baking* and *The Vegan Table*, and is the founder of Compassionate Cooks (www.compassionatecooks.com), an organization whose mission is to empower people to make informed food choices, to inspire people to live according to their values of compassion and health, and to debunk myths about veganism and animal rights.

A sought-after and inspiring public speaker on the spiritual, social, and practical aspects of a compassionate lifestyle, Colleen focuses her work on debunking myths about veganism and animal rights and empowering people to make informed food choices. She has appeared on the Food Network and is a columnist for *VegNews Magazine* and a contributor to National Public Radio. She lives in Oakland, California with her husband and two cats.

INDEX

RECIPE INDEX